Supporting Children with Dyslexia

Garry Squires and Sally McKeown

Practical approaches for teachers and parents

QUESTIONS
PUBLISHING

The *Questions Publishing Company* Ltd
Birmingham
2003

The Questions Publishing Company Ltd
Leonard House, 321 Bradford Street, Digbeth, Birmingham B5 6ET

© The Questions Publishing Company Ltd 2003

First published in 2003

ISBN: 1-84190-085-0

Editorial team: Linda Evans
                       Amanda Greenley

Design by: James Davies
Illustrations by: Iqbal Aslam

Cover photograph by: Amanda Greenley

With thanks to staff and children at Leasowes Community College.

Printed in the UK

Contents

Introduction

Dyslexia is a term used to describe people who have specific difficulties in learning to read, write and spell. It may be neurological in origin and can often have associated difficulties with memory and sequential thinking. Dyslexia is not new – it has been around for as long as people have endeavoured to read and write and has been recognised as a difficulty in developing these skills since it was first described by James Kerr and Pringle Morgan in 1896 (see box below). Likewise, compulsory schooling has been around for well over a hundred years and has always had an emphasis on literacy – potentially disadvantaging dyslexic pupils. It is likely that every present-day classroom will have four or five children who have a degree of dyslexia.

Pringle Morgan described a case of a 14-year-old boy, Percy F. He described him as a *"bright and intelligent boy, quick at games, and in no way inferior to others of his age"*.

He went on to describe Percy's unexpected difficulty with reading: *"His great difficulty has been – and is now – his ability to learn to read. This inability is so remarkable, and so pronounced, that I have no doubt it is due to some congenital defect"*.

Pringle Morgan highlighted that this was not due to poor teaching. *"He has been at school or under tutors since he was 7 years old, and the greatest efforts have been made to teach him to read, but, in spite of this laborious and persistent training, he can only with difficulty spell out words of one syllable."*

He gives an example of Percy's spelling: ***"Now, you word me wale I spin if. Calfuly winder the sturng rond the Pag"***. [Now, you watch me while I spin it. Carefully winding the string round the peg.]

Morgan, W. M. (1896) A Case of Congenital Word Blindness *The British Medical Journal.*

What do you do with dyslexic children?

There are plenty of books about dyslexia and well-structured teaching packs that focus on the remediation of difficulties. But not much is written about the day-to-day work that goes on in mainstream classrooms or about how parents can help. This book sets out to address this issue by providing an understanding of what it is like to be dyslexic and giving ideas that focus on the solutions to problems that may be encountered.

Inclusion of dyslexic children

The term 'dyslexia' evokes anxiety and uncertainty for some teachers who hear it being used to describe a child with whom they have contact. Equally, parents worry that if their child is dyslexic then they can only be taught successfully by a 'specialist' teacher (who has a qualification in teaching dyslexic children). Anecdotal examples of this from an Educational Psychologist include:

"One child had made tremendous progress on small step targets for literacy set on his Individual Education Programme (IEP), yet his class teacher continued to comment in a negative way about how he was not able to do any better in class. A very successful remedial programme had led to an increase in literacy skills yet somehow this was not seen as helpful to the teacher. What could be done to lead to an improvement in performance in class? How could the class teacher be helped to support the child more effectively in day-to-day classroom work?"

"Work with a child with reading difficulties had resulted in Statutory Assessment being undertaken and a Statement of Special Educational Needs had been produced offering support. A few days later the parent telephoned me and was quite concerned; her son's class teacher had made a comment that she did not know anything about dyslexia."

(Squires, 2001c)

The Code of Practice for Special Educational Needs (DfES, 2001) provides guidance for working with pupils who have a wide range of educational needs including dyslexia. The Code of Practice promotes inclusion and sets out an expectation that children with special educational needs will normally have their needs met in a mainstream school and have access to a broad and balanced National Curriculum. In terms of dyslexia this means that schools need to understand what it is like to be dyslexic and what can be done to facilitate learning for these pupils. A number of local education authorities have embarked on raising awareness of dyslexia in schools to help them become more 'dyslexia friendly' with accreditation from the British Dyslexia Association.

Teachers are skilled professionals who already have a range of strategies that are helpful to dyslexic children. By constantly updating their resources and seeking support from SENCos (Special Educational Needs Coordinators) and outside specialists, they successfully deal with an ever-increasing range of diagnosed difficulties in their classrooms. One role for this book is to help teachers reflect on, and become more skilled in dealing with, individual differences by considering alternative approaches to enhancing their teaching skills. It has been argued that reflection leads to greater awareness of what 'constitutes appropriate pedagogic practice' (Kullman, 1998) and encourages personal development (Bulsrode and Hunt, 2000). Conversation is seen as an important way of making sense of teaching experiences, and as a means of exchanging ideas and new ways to act in the classroom (Stanulis and Russell, 2000). This book is presented as a catalyst for reflection, discussion and development as well as being a source of ideas and strategies.

Some of this material has previously been given in booklet form to teachers and has enabled them to consider how best to meet individual needs and help dyslexic pupils to achieve. Such an approach helps to contribute towards an inclusive ethos of dyslexia friendly schools. As one teacher said:

"Using these ideas has helped me recognise what I do already, it has given me some new ideas...it has helped me feel more confident and it has helped my pupil be more confident in class."

Figure 1: Changes in teacher confidence ratings when given information about dyslexia (Squires, 2001a)

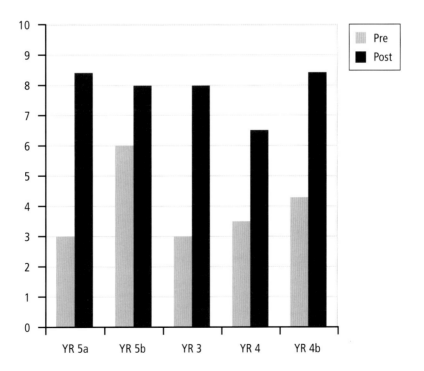

Making a graduated response

The Code of Practice recognises that there is a continuum of special educational needs. The dyslexia spectrum runs from pupils with severe dyslexia, who find print very intimidating and need a high level of support, to those who are able to record their ideas in writing but whose spelling is somewhat idiosyncratic. This means that teachers will have to notice what children find difficult and then respond by modifying their teaching – this is the principle of early intervention. The responsibility for meeting a child's special educational needs rests with the class teacher. Advice may be sought from other specialists or from the SENCo. This allows the school to make a graduated response – those children who need the most help are able to receive it while those who need the least are encouraged to work independently.

The Code of Practice sets out three levels of support:

● *School Action* – the steps that the class teacher, SENCo and school can take to provide support.
● *School Action Plus* – the school seeks additional advice from outside agencies (advisory teachers, speech and language therapists, occupational therapists, educational psychologists, etc).
● *Statement of Special Educational Needs* – the child's needs are considered to be long term and complex and requiring more than has been provided at School Action and School Action Plus.

Schools can request Statutory Assessment, and best practice is contained in the Code of Practice Toolkit section called 'Writing Advice'. The LEA will usually request all relevant records, including evidence that IEPs have been designed and implemented in attempting to meet the needs of the child. The information will include records of the pupil's progress in the National Curriculum and any standardised test results. The LEA will then decide whether or not to proceed with the assessment, which will involve an Educational Psychologist and a medical report as well as input from any other agencies involved with the child (e.g. social services). Parents' views have to be considered too. The issuing of a Statement should take a maximum of six months and it must then be reviewed annually and at school transfer time. Statements issued to dyslexic children usually specify a certain amount of specialist support and can trigger special consideration in exams, such as extra time or the help of an amanuensis.

There is currently a move away from Statementing however, as many think it a bureaucratic and costly process that diverts energy and money away from children. This means that many LEAs will be looking for alternative ways of providing support to dyslexic children, such as improving the skills of mainstream teachers and teaching assistants. It is generally referred to as 'capacity building' – improving the whole school by increasing teaching skills. This is the principle behind 'dyslexia friendly' initiatives and behind this book.

Parents as equal partners

The Code of Practice values the role of parents as equal in status to that of teachers and other professionals. It recognises that parents have a vital part to play in contributing to how their children's educational needs can be met.

● Parents are experts about what it is like to live with their children. Parents can contribute important information about the problems facing the child at home – perhaps the dyslexic child struggles for hours to complete homework that is expected to take other children in his or her class 20 minutes. Parents will have developed strategies for supporting the child's organisation or for checking that they understand instructions when they are told to do something. Parents will know many of the child's strengths and weaknesses and can help by sharing with staff their solutions to day-to-day problems that exist at home, which can be transferred into school.
● Parents will have personal resources and time that they can commit to supporting the child. These will depend on:
  ● how much patience a person has,
  ● how well they can read or write,
  ● how good their rapport is with their children,
  ● how well they are able to explain things,
  ● the extent to which they can encourage and motivate the child,
  ● how anxious they feel about their child's progress, and
  ● how well they are able to deal with the child's worries and frustrations.
● There is some evidence to suggest that dyslexia might run in families. If this is the case, the parents might themselves have faced and solved the problems now facing the child. Questions such as 'What works for you?' or 'How do you remember things?' may provide valuable insights into finding ways of supporting the child.
● Parents can help with monitoring and can carry out simple remedial programmes under the guidance of the class teacher.

Many schools encourage parents to participate through regular meetings with teaching staff and/or support staff. The Code of Practice recommends that when a child has an identified special educational need, parents and school should review progress together at least twice a year (one time might be part of a normal parental consultation evening). Some schools run courses to help parents develop specific skills to support their children.

Summary

- Dyslexic children are found in mainstream classrooms and it is expected that they will be included in a broad and balanced curriculum. The responsibility for their teaching lies with their class teacher.
- Schools and parents want access to information to help them understand the needs of dyslexic children and how they can be supported in mainstream classes.
- Teachers already have a range of skills and expertise and can draw upon more from support agencies and outside specialists.
- Parents have a valuable contribution to make and schools have a responsibility to involve parents as equal partners.
- There is a continuum of dyslexia and a graduated response can be made to help the child become an independent learner.
- There needs to be a focus on solutions so that the presenting problems are not seen as being insurmountable.

Definitions and Challenges

Teachers frequently encounter children with reading and spelling difficulties and need to consider how best to support them across the curriculum. A survey involving over fifty schools in ten local education authorities found evidence of good practice when looking at how pupils with Statements for specific learning difficulties were progressing in reading, spelling and writing (Ofsted, 1999). However, when teachers are asked about how confident they feel about teaching dyslexic children, they do not always respond as would be expected. They seem to see dyslexic children as having greatly different needs to other 'common or garden' poor readers or poor spellers. Teachers were asked to describe children with reading and writing difficulties and they were asked to define dyslexia. Their responses are tabled below:

Table 1: Constructs used by teachers (Squires, 2001a)

Dyslexia Concept	Overlap	Literacy Difficulty Concept
● many aspects/traits ← → single difficulty	● trouble with reading, writing and spelling	● lack of experience of reading
● different types of dyslexia	● not being able to decode symbols	● poor phonological skills
● problems with rote learning		● poor behaviour due to frustration
● confusion with textual information		● low confidence
● sequencing difficulties		● dependent learning style/teacher reliant
● intelligence		● poor quality of work
● neurological processing difficulty		● slow
● good oral/aural but poor written		● thinks everything is wrong
● poor concentration		● hard to motivate
		● restricted vocabulary when writing

There appears very little overlap between the two concepts being constructed by teachers. Maybe this is because there are many definitions of dyslexia, each one emphasising slightly different features or views about the nature and causes of the difficulties. This leads to some confusion and then teachers become uncertain about what to do.

The single factor that unifies the different definitions of dyslexia is a weakness in reading and spelling. Differences in failure to learn to read or spell adequately can be explained by a number of hypotheses:

- *phonological deficit hypothesis* – difficulty with decoding sound or spoken language inhibits development of normal spelling or reading;
- *visual processing deficit hypothesis* – difficulty with decoding visual information inhibits development of normal reading or spelling;
- *transient magnocellular deficit hypothesis* – difficulty with responding to rapid changes of sound or visual information interferes with normal reading and spelling;
- *developmental delay hypothesis* – there is a general immaturity in neurological development and this means that reading and spelling develop along normal lines but much more slowly;
- *central executive control dysfunction hypothesis* – integration of information from the visual and verbal pathways is incomplete and this inhibits reading and spelling development;
- *automaticity impairment hypothesis* – fluency in decoding textual information is impaired, making reading and spelling more arduous.

The full details of these different hypotheses are beyond the scope of this book. Suffice it to say that these explanations arise partly from the starting perspective of the researchers and the way in which they define dyslexia and select participants for their investigations. However:

- each hypothesis is supported by research evidence,
- different parts of the brain are implicated,
- a range of cognitive profiles are evident when test scores are examined, and
- developmental processes influence ocular stability and control, speech production and phonological awareness, motor control and co-ordination, and ability to respond to the level of textual information.

This leads to the view that dyslexia is a collection of conditions characterised by poor reading and/or poor spelling with a number of cognitive processes involved that produce different patterns of strengths and weaknesses in different children (Squires, 2003).

Different definitions of dyslexia

The working party of the British Psychological Society (1999) have offered a broad definition of dyslexia:

"Dyslexia is evident when accurate and fluent word reading and/or spelling develops very incompletely or with great difficulty. This focuses on literacy learning at the 'word level' and implies that the problem is severe and persistent despite appropriate learning opportunities. It provides the basis for a staged process of assessment through teaching."

The definition emphasises:

- a lack of accuracy in reading or spelling,
- a lack of fluency when reading or spelling,
- a problem at the 'word level' of the National Literacy Strategy,
- the need for appropriate teaching,
- the severity and persistence of the difficulties, and
- an interaction between teaching and learning.

The definition is not exclusive and this means that any child with literacy difficulties that are severe and persistent and not responsive to well-structured, frequently provided remedial teaching could be considered as being dyslexic.

The definition offered is not universally accepted amongst psychologists or teachers, with some preferring aspects of other definitions of dyslexia. Some suggest that dyslexia is organic in origin. Many definitions include an *unexpected* inability of the child to develop literacy skills despite good teaching (e.g. Brooks and Weeks, 2000, suggest that discrepancies should remain a part of assessment packages). Some definitions focus on the linguistic aspects (e.g. Heaton and Winterson, 1996; Rack, 1994). Others offer a definition that takes into account a core problem and a collection of associated difficulties (e.g. Turner, 1997). Some definitions describe the core problems as being related to how the brain is able to make repeated actions fluent by making them automatic (e.g. Nicholson and Fawcett, 1995, 1999).

These other definitions outline a range of associated factors:

- difficulties with short term memory capacity,
- difficulties with working memory,
- phonological difficulties (e.g. difficulty with sound awareness),
- visual difficulties (see page 10),
- perceptual difficulties,
- an unexpected difference between performance in some areas and performance in literacy,
- a slow speed in noticing, processing and responding to information,
- poor organisational skills and planning skills,
- a lack of fluency,
- difficulty with automaticity.

For some children there are additional difficulties. They may:

- become over-reliant on adult support,
- become reluctant to try, even when the task is well within their capability,
- have low self-esteem and feelings of low self-worth,
- avoid academic tasks, particularly those involving reading or writing,
- develop emotional and behavioural difficulties.

Visual dyslexia

In any class there are likely to be two or three children who have a visual problem that stops them acquiring the skills needed for reading. When this is more than a straightforward physiological problem (e.g. myopia or short-sightedness) it may warrant further investigation.

When we read, our eyes have to do a number of things:

- see the words clearly and transmit the image to the brain. Good readers can work with quite blurred images but poor sight handicaps beginner readers.
- work together so that both are focused on the same point. Some learners have an eye condition that results in the print moving around on the page. They may also be more aware of the white spaces between words, and find that instead of taking in a range of letters or words at a glance, they only take in one or two letters so they never get a sense of the whole word or word shape.
- stay focused on close work
- move in a controlled way. Pupils may have a tracking difficulty that affects their ability to move the eyes along a line, and onto the next line without losing their place.

Recognising visual dyslexia

Look out for children:

- with a history of eye problems,
- suffering with headaches,
- rubbing their eyes,
- 'squinting' to try to improve clarity of print,
- closing one eye when reading,
- holding a book very near, or at arm's length, when reading,
- laying their head on the desk when writing,
- with photo-phobia – a dislike of the light (they might screw up their eyes),
- who have difficulty moving from one line to another (they may use a finger or marker to follow the line),
- with poor visual discrimination,
- complaining that words or letters won't 'keep still',
- 'guessing' the ends of words or letters.

If you notice these signs and the child is a poor reader, you need to suggest to the parents or carers that they seek advice. Quite often a visit to an ordinary optician is not enough as they are not specialists in this area. Some chains of opticians are now training staff to recognise and treat this problem but provision is patchy. Parents may find that the best route is via their family doctor who can refer the child to a specialist, such as an optometrist who can test for eye stability.

There is a whole battery of assessments that can be performed to identify the problem. Obviously the first step is a sight test to see if the child is long- or short-sighted. Long sight can make reading very uncomfortable. Other tests might include an examination of the eye to see if it is healthy and a check to see if the eye muscles work properly.

An optometrist may also check for:

● Pattern glare problems caused by contrast. These are exacerbated by the fact that most text is presented as black print on white paper.
● Fixation difficulties where the child cannot consistently focus on a word.
● Tracking abnormalities.
● Fusional disturbances where the words jumble or move.

Other tests might include:

● *Opthalmokinetic Assessment,* which assesses the eye tracking and may be used to predict whether a child is likely to have reading difficulties. The child may be asked to look at light stimulants. The way a child's eyes register and process information may indicate specific neurological disorders. A dyslexic will have a harder time focusing on the lights, as well as concentration problems.
● *The Dunlop Test,* which identifies unstable binocularity. Usually treatment involves covering one eye to establish stable fixation.
● *The Irlen Assessment,* which establishes whether coloured overlays, tinted lenses or contact lenses help the individual. Usually pupils start with a trial set of lenses, designed to be worn all the time.

Some reading difficulties are attributed to unstable eye dominance, which can affect the ability to scan from left to right. Such individuals confuse direction, reversing letters such as 'b' and 'd', and have difficulty with the order and sequence of numbers.

Specialists may recommend treatments that range from putting a patch over one eye when reading to correctional contact lenses, eye exercises, coloured overlays or Irlen lenses.

Positive traits in dyslexia

Dyslexia is a condition that generally leads to people thinking about limitations and the way the condition stops children from accessing the curriculum or recording their ideas. This way of framing dyslexia can be damaging to children – it wears away their self-esteem and always focuses on their short-comings.

However, having dyslexia can enable some young people to develop amazing talents. This may be because they are able to process certain types of information more effectively, or it may be because they develop compensatory strategies.

An example of a compensatory strategy found in some dyslexics is a very good verbal memory. This comes about because teachers normally support children during class discussions by writing information on the board. If you are dyslexic and cannot read the information easily, then you have no choice but to remember it. This seems to develop memory skills for verbal information.

One strength reported by many dyslexics is increased artistic ability. Perhaps because they are less able to communicate verbally or in writing, some dyslexics develop their artistic skills as a means of expressing themselves.

Teachers and parents can help dyslexic children search for their talents and strengths and encourage them to develop those areas of interest at which they do well.

Famous people who are thought to have been dyslexic are often cited in newspapers, examples from *The Guardian* (Nov. 98) include:

- Leonardo de Vinci

- Hans Christian Anderson

- Auguste Rodin

- Thomas Edison

- Winston Churchill

- Albert Einstein

- Richard Rogers

- Tom Cruise

Whether some of the earlier people in the list would be defined as dyslexic by today's standards remains unclear. But the message is important – dyslexic type difficulties should not be a barrier to doing great things.

The challenge for teachers

Learning and teaching are reciprocal and occur as a social interaction in which the more competent teacher structures the learning environment and tasks of the less competent pupil. This reframing of teaching and learning means that often children's learning difficulties are seen as teachers' teaching difficulties. Teaching is viewed as involving more than *delivering* a curriculum, what requires some thought is how the teacher can help the learner to access the curriculum and record ideas.

The model of intervention changes from attempting to improve children's performance through remedial teaching, to inviting the teacher to engage in a reflection of their teaching strategies. How will the teacher respond to the child's needs while covering the breadth of content of the curriculum? How can challenging work be presented to a bright child who has difficulty accessing text or recording their ideas in writing?

Schools are expected to include dyslexic pupils in the mainstream of classroom activities. This means that teachers will need to notice differences in pupil performance and respond to them. They will need to know what to look for and to have a range of strategies that allow effective responses. Effective support can be provided without having to resort to Statements of SEN, but may involve LEA support agencies and the efficient deployment of LEA resources.

Individual Education Plans continue to focus on remedial education with clearly defined SMART (Specific, Measurable, Achievable, Relevant, Timed) targets. There are plenty of packages available to help teachers address remediation. What is often missing is a statement on the IEP about how the child will be supported through the adaptation of the learning environment or teaching strategies used.

Perhaps IEPs need to be widened in their scope to include specific classroom management and support techniques. This would then prompt class teachers and subject teachers when thinking about planning their lessons. It could also prompt parents into thinking about things they could do to help their child during the day and with homework. (See pages 29–34.)

The next chapter invites you to think about how children with reading and spelling difficulties can be supported on a day-to-day basis in the classroom, doing their normal work and being included in the mainstream curriculum. The case studies on pages 14 and 15 exemplify some of these children.

Summary

● There are many different definitions of dyslexia – each emphasises something slightly different. This can make the term dyslexia seem unsuitable as a diagnostic term. However, all agree that the term implies a significant difficulty in reading and spelling.

● Some definitions acknowledge that dyslexia is a much wider problem that interferes with other areas of life as well as learning in school. What is certain is that no two dyslexic children are the same – each has slightly different presenting difficulties. Each child also has a different range of strengths that can be developed.

● Somehow, teachers and parents have to notice these difficulties and respond to them. This book explores some of the solutions that can be tried.

Five case studies

Charles

Charles attends his local secondary school. When there are class discussions, he seems bright – always keen to answer the teacher's questions and he has lots of ideas.

At parents' evenings his teachers often comment on the extent of his general knowledge – but also on his lack of ability to 'get anything down on paper'. Homework is never done; he never has the right equipment for lessons.

When he does manage to produce something it is untidy, poorly set out and his ideas are poorly structured. His spelling is described as 'weird' and he takes an age to read though questions. His test results in class do not reflect what he can do. Some teachers think he is lazy.

John

John is a Year 5 pupil – he's in trouble again. Every lesson his teacher has to tell him to stop wandering around and to sit in his place! As soon as the class starts work he's off – chatting to this one, borrowing a rubber off that one – or just sharpening his pencil. He must get though several pencils in a week!

Ahmed

Ahmed is superb at art – his drawing of the school is up on the wall in the Head teacher's office and some of his collage work was displayed in the library. He is popular with his peers and was chosen to be the captain of the school football team.

His literacy is not so good. In his Key Stage 2 SATs he managed to get Level 2 overall for English, while in Maths he achieved a Level 5.

Julie

Julie is eight years old. She has a history of ear infections and 'glue ear'. Her speech is unclear and indistinct with sounds mixed up. She has seen a Speech and Language Therapist and things are improving.

In school, her reading is well behind the rest of the class. Her knowledge of letter sounds is incomplete. She gets upset because her reading book is not the same as everyone else's. At home, reading is a real battle – tears and tantrums are common.

Callum

Callum's mum is worried. Despite his poor reading and writing, he has done well in his primary school. This has been because his teacher knows him well and has been very supportive. But in September, he will transfer to the High School. "*What will happen to him then? He won't be able to keep up with the work and he will get lost in such a big school.*"

I wonder how he'll cope?

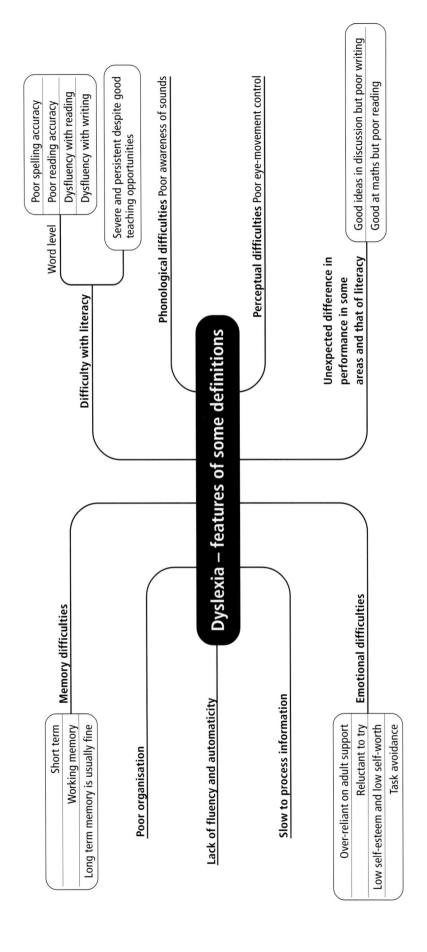

Dyslexia – features of some definitions

Difficulty with literacy

Word level
- Poor spelling accuracy
- Poor reading accuracy
- Dysfluency with reading
- Dysfluency with writing

Severe and persistent despite good teaching opportunities

Phonological difficulties Poor awareness of sounds

Perceptual difficulties Poor eye-movement control

Unexpected difference in performance in some areas and that of literacy
- Good ideas in discussion but poor writing
- Good at maths but poor reading

Memory difficulties
- Short term
- Working memory
- Long term memory is usually fine

Poor organisation

Lack of fluency and automaticity

Slow to process information

Emotional difficulties
- Over-reliant on adult support
- Reluctant to try
- Low self-esteem and low self-worth
- Task avoidance

Identifying Strengths and Weaknesses

It is all too easy to emphasise the negative aspects of dyslexia and unwittingly contribute to a child's feelings of inadequacy and failure. While assessing strengths and weaknesses can be useful – for pupil, parents and teachers – it is important to remember to 'accentuate the positive' at all times and remind pupils of what they CAN do as well as identifying and addressing the tasks that present difficulties for them.

A good starting place to protect children's self-esteem is to list all the things they do well. This can be done using notes, key words, drawings or photographs. Celebration charts, merit points and certificates can be used judiciously to reward effort and boost self-confidence.

A great deal of celebration in schools is to do with neat presentation of work, well-written text and expressive reading aloud. But there are many other attributes/skills/actions worthy of recognition:

- Being polite/kind/thoughtful/helpful/patient/persistent.
- Being good at art, music, model-making, cookery, sport.
- Keeping a secret, remembering something, taking care of animals, befriending 'the new boy'.

Checklist

The different definitions of dyslexia suggest points that could be included on a checklist. When completing the list, remember that children are developing all the time and think about how well a particular pupil compares with others of the same age. This is important since a child aged 18 months would show all of the signs of dyslexia on the DfEE checklist for primary school teachers (DfEE, undated).

The checklist is constructed from the main definitions and phrased in a positive way so that you can think about what the child *can* do. Several columns have been added so that you can record progress over time.

2

Name: Date of birth:	Rating scale **Blank** = can't do yet **1** = can do with help **2** = can do independently **3** = can do well			
Date:				
Speed of processing				
Speaks quickly and fluently				
Reads quickly				
Writes quickly				
Solves problems quickly				
Memory				
Remembers three things when told to bring them from another room				
Remembers a telephone number				
Can relate events that have happened days ago				
Remembers to do things that are planned				
Retains new knowledge				
Can recall address				
Retains new words that are read				
Retains new spellings				
Independence				
Ties shoelaces				
Dresses self				
Reading				
Can tell if two words sound the same (rhyme)				
Recognises all of the letter sounds or names				
Can sort out similar looking letters (e.g. 'b' from 'd', 'u' from 'n')				
Has strategies for attempting new words				
Manages to read the small linking words (e.g. a, and, the, of, it, is)				
Can keep track of place and position when reading				

Writing

Writes name unaided				
Writes numbers in correct orientation				
Makes own notes following discussion				
Writes with few crossings out				
Writes in a cursive style				

Spelling

Spells words consistently				
Spellings make sense				
Can recognise when an error has been made				
85% or more of spellings are correct				

Co-ordination

Rides a bike				
Has a clear preference or handedness				
Knows which is right and left				
Produces well-formed letters				
Is able to produce clear drawings				
Holds pencil correctly				

Organisation

Sets out written work well				
Has an even space at the start of each line next to the margin or page edge				
Remembers to bring pencil case, books, PE kit to school				

Behaviour

Is able to sit still and concentrate on non-literacy tasks				
Is able to sit still and concentrate on literacy tasks				
Chooses to read				
Chooses to write				
Participates in all aspects of lesson				
Keen to go to school				
Keen to go to lessons				

2

SUPPORTING CHILDREN

Reading and spelling ages

There will be a range of reading abilities and spelling abilities within any classroom just as there will be a range of heights and weights. To some extent, reading and spelling achievement as measured by tests will depend upon the particular test used. Such assessments can be useful however, especially when shared with all staff who come into contact with a dyslexic pupil, as a way of reminding them of his limitations. If teachers know that a pupil has a reading age of 7.0 in his first year of secondary school, they will realise that he is going to need a lot of support in using a text book that requires a reading age of 11.0. There are instances however, where detailed testing is carried out by the SENCo and support staff, as a means of gathering diagnostic information and monitoring individual progress, but outcomes are not shared with subject teachers.

Reading and spelling ages of children considered in the average range for reading

Different reading and spelling tests give different age scores for the same child. Most people consider that an average child would have a reading and spelling age equal to their chronological age and worry if the test shows that they are below this level. However, there is a spread around 'the average' with the normal distribution curve showing that most children have a reading and spelling age either just below or above their chronological age.

If children's test scores are put in order so they go from the lowest to the highest, then the child's rank order position can be obtained. This goes from 1 to 100, and is referred to as a centile score. Statistically, the average is considered to go from the 16th centile position to the 84th centile position.

Table 2 shows the ages obtained on three common tests used by psychologists to measure reading. They show the age of children who are performing at the 16th centile level (i.e. at the bottom end of the 'average' band). The Code of Practice for Special Educational Needs suggests that remediation is only necessary if a child is not making adequate progress and is falling below the majority of their peers. The spread in ability gets wider as children get older. Being just over one year behind is seen as a cause for concern at age 7, but by the age of 16 a pupil would be 3 to 4 years behind before attracting the same concern.

Table 2

Age of child	BAS-II	WORD	NARA-II
5.0–6.0 is below the minimum age measurable on the test selected.			
7.0	5.9 to 5.10	6.3	6.1
8.0	6.10	7.0	6.7
9.0	7.10	7.9	7.3
10.0	8.3	8.9	7.10
11.0	8.9 to 8.10	8.9	8.6
12.0	9.10 to 9.11	9.3	9.1
13.0	10.10 to 10.11	9.6	9.6
14.0	11.5 to 11.7	10.3	Not suitable for children over 12.11
15.0	12.5 to 12.8	10.9	
16.0	13.6 to 13.8	11.9	

Classroom observations

The Code of Practice for Special Educational Needs places an emphasis on teachers noticing children's difficulties and then adjusting their teaching accordingly. This means that teachers need to be on the lookout for potential difficulties that the dyslexic child might have and then respond with a suitable strategy to ameliorate the difficulties.

The kinds of questions that might be helpful are:

- What am I asking the pupils to do?
- What parts of this task can this particular pupil do without any help?
- What might they be able to do if they work with a more competent peer?
- What could they do in a different way?
- How have they done similar things before?
- How might I be able to break the task down so that they can achieve success using added structure?
- Where might an adult be needed to help them? In what way?

Chapter 3, Classroom Settings and Supportive Strategies, provides a long list of suggestions for helping dyslexic children.

Noting things that help

Dyslexia has been found to 'run in families'. Often, if a child is diagnosed as dyslexic, then one of their parents or grandparents also had difficulty with learning to read or spell. This provides a useful way of finding things that might work with the child. Ask the adult questions like: 'What helped you?', 'How did you solve such and such a problem?', 'How do you…?'

Parents can take time to note what seems to help at home. Equally, when a child is going to transfer to a new class, the existing teacher can make a note of things that have helped.

Analysing spelling patterns

Some checklists include the item 'bizarre spelling' and we often consider some children's spelling as being very idiosyncratic. It seems to make sense to them but is not accepted in English. However, an understanding of how spelling skills develop allows us to look beyond this framing.

As children's spelling skills start to emerge they move through a set pattern of learning. Their accuracy gradually increases and when they make mistakes, their attempts become more and more like the target word. The types of mistakes that they make suggest particular types of processing difficulties or particular types of processing strengths. Understanding these strengths and weaknesses can help in deciding the kinds of approaches to use in remediation or the features of particular spellings to emphasise during classroom work.

Treiman (1997) presents a model of spelling development that focuses on the phonological development of spelling. In her paper she describes dyslexic spelling as being similar to that produced by younger children. This has been expanded here to include visual errors (adapted from Squires, 2003):

Pre-spelling

Early spellings start off as being simple representations of words – scribblings that are recognisable as being different from the child's drawings. Perhaps the marks are smaller or they travel in a line. The child is playing at writing and perhaps copying what parents or older siblings seem to be doing. Big objects tend to get big words.

Syllabic-grapheme

By reception stage, children are starting to learn that letters convey meaning. At this stage they may expect a single letter to represent a syllable.

As spelling develops, children learn how to put letters together in a certain order to correctly represent the word they want to use. Spelling errors can be classified as either being a verbal-phonological error or as being a visuo-spatial error. Some spellings might seem to belong to both categories.

Verbal errors made at the phoneme-grapheme stage

● *Phonemic representation* – there is increasing consistency of letter use to represent the sounds that the child hears, e.g. 'eat' is written as 'it' (i/t).
● *Consonant omission* – the child has difficulties when the sound is represented by more than one letter. Typical errors include 'drik' for 'drink', 'cod' for 'cold' or 'wom' for 'warm'.
● *Vowel omission* – the vowels are not needed to write the sounds in words and are sometimes missed out, e.g. 'hotl' for 'hotel', 'hr' for 'her'.
● *Immature speech patterns are evident in spelling* – examples include saying 'jr' instead of 'dr' (e.g. 'jragon') or 'ch' instead of 'tr'.
● *Phonologically plausible but orthographic errors* – particular letter reversals are more likely than others because children remember what the sound is.

Visual-spatial errors

● *Sequence errors* – the letters are present but in the wrong order, e.g. 'wtiring'.
● *Addition of extra letters* – extra letters are added to the word, e.g. 'offten'.
● *Omission of letters* – letters are left out, e.g. 'stiker'.
● *Orientation of letters* – letters are confused with similar looking letters, e.g. u/n, w/m, b/d/p/q.
● *Form* – confusions are related to the form of the letter, e.g. n/h, i/j, i/l, a/e/o. This includes gestalt errors, for example perceiving

closure on 'i' to make 'l' or on 'c' to make 'o'.

- *Global errors* – the word has the right start and right end and is about the right length.

Morphemic spelling

The child starts to take account of meaning and etymology. For example 'heal' and 'health' both carry the same meaning and have the same morpheme 'heal'. Errors now involve selecting the wrong morpheme.

Some spellings cannot be easily assigned to just one category and may need to be placed in more than one category. But a diagnostic count can be made of the types of errors made and this can guide the next step in remediation. The chart on page 24 allows this to be done.

Remedial programmes

For pupils with significant problems, part of a school's response is often the instigation of some sort of structured remedial programme. This can be an opportunity to focus on specific areas of difficulty, often outside the normal classroom situation and away from the attentions of curious peers.

For children with difficulties severe enough to require a Statement of Special Educational Needs it has been found that:

- progress is better when children's needs are identified early and Statements carry specialist support,
- better progress is made when additional focused teaching is provided,
- good progress in reading is linked to a highly structured programme of teaching often involving a multisensory approach (a recommendation was made that this should be available earlier on and before a Statement was required), and
- effective programmes go beyond merely hearing the child read and include teaching the use of context cues; discussion of the content to aid understanding; systematic teaching of word groups and the sounds of clusters of letters.
(Ofsted,1999)

These features can be applied equally of course, to pupils who are receiving additional support at the *School Action* or *School Action Plus* stage.

A feature of many good remedial programmes is repetition and over-learning of materials that the child finds difficult to learn. Well-designed programmes involve daily practice often lasting only ten to fifteen minutes. This is because memory is more efficient when practice is distributed across several learning periods rather than massed into one learning session. It has other important gains too:

- *The child expects the learning to take place; the routine helps to*

Morphemic			
Visual	Global		
	Form		
	Orientation		
	Sequence/addition/omission		
	Closure		
Phonological	Orthographic (phonologically plausible)		
	Phoneme-grapheme	Immature speech pattern evident in spelling	
		Vowel omission	
		Final consonant omission	
		Phonemic representation (one sound per syllable)	
	Syllabic-grapheme		
	Pre-spelling		

prepare him for the activity.

- The activities tend to be fast-paced and this reduces the opportunities for attention wandering and concentration waning.
- Short duration tasks are easier to fit into the busy schedule of a school or the domestic demands placed upon a busy parent.

Precision teaching is a good example of distributed practice and may include exercises such as a one-minute daily exercise to see how many 'b's and 'd's the child can successfully read from a grid of randomly presented 'b's and 'd's. This type of exercise provides the child with instant feedback and always focuses on success. Progress can be easily monitored by keeping a daily count or by using a weekly probe sheet.

Learning stages

Learning progresses through well defined stages:

1. *Unknown skills and knowledge* – learning has not taken place.
2. *Acquisition* – the child is just starting to learn, getting it right on some days but not others.
3. *Mastery learning* – the child gets it right all of the time in the learning situation, but does not apply the new knowledge consistently in the classroom.
4. *Generalisation* – the child gets it right all of the time, in the learning situation and beyond.

Sometimes children fail in teaching programmes because the pace of the programme is too quick and is focused on the teaching materials rather than the child's learning. The materials move on to the next skill or item of knowledge while the child is left at the acquisition stage. Without consolidation they will not master the skill or knowledge and will not be able to apply it in their everyday work. This is sometimes compounded when programmes are designed in which each piece of new learning builds upon learning that is expected to have taken place in earlier parts of the programme.

Good programmes need to take into account the fact that memory fades and needs renewal of the 'memory trace' to sustain learning. Some teaching assistants ask the child to recall one thing he has learnt at the end of each lesson and ask the same question at the beginning of the next lesson. This reinforces recall and, by saying it out loud, it helps to fix the idea in the mind. Some intervention programmes incorporate interleaved learning in which old material is interleaved with the new. Once learning has reached generalisation level, learning is sustained through daily use and practice. At this level, interleaved learning is not necessary.

When selecting a remedial programme we need to somehow take the child's classroom-based learning into the remedial situation and vice versa. One way of doing this is to start with the mistakes that the child makes with literacy, e.g. using miscue analysis in reading. The teacher could start by looking at the child's writing and doing some targeted

Computer programs from CALSC have been used successfully in some schools. *Mastering Memory* is a general program for children to identify their strengths and to help them develop strategies for memorising information (www.calsc.co.uk). Some children seem to know what works for them and have good methods in place; others need direct teaching if they are to learn how to learn.

marking to find the three most common errors made by the child in spelling. This would then allow remedial teaching to focus on the types of errors made. Progress during remedial work then feeds back into improved accuracy in class work. Positive feedback about this will increase the child's self-confidence and their view of themselves as a successful independent learner. If the teacher continues to target-mark the words identified earlier then there is feedback about daily performance and a systematic way of monitoring the extent of generalisation. Generalisation can be further supported through the class teacher looking for opportunities to teach the spelling throughout the day. For example:

- drawing attention to the spelling rule in whole class work,
- checking the child's application of the spelling 'in passing' through the lesson,
- teaching the spelling rule and reminding of the spelling rule through group work or whole class work, or in visiting the child to provide individual support,
- having reminders of the target spelling rules displayed around the room in a variety of formats, and
- playing 'spot the mistake' by deliberately making the mistake in board work and then asking the class to spot the mistake and say how the word could be corrected.

Making good links between support workers (teaching assistants, specialist advisory teachers, SENCo) and the class teacher or subject teachers will maximise learning and generalisation. For instance if the remedial programme is focusing on breaking words down into syllables as a word-attack strategy when reading, then this can be extended into the classroom:

- When the child gets stuck on a word when reading a class text, the teacher or teaching assistant can take the child through the stages of breaking the word down and then blending the different segments produced. The teacher comes along and asks the child questions to prompt the actions required, rather than simply telling the child what the word is. If the steps are too large then the adult can break the steps down even further. The child is then able to succeed in the strategy with the adult's help and is learning in the *zone of proximal development*. The emphasis is on the child succeeding and this has a positive effect on the child's self-esteem.
- The class teacher can use the strategy to model the process in whole class teaching for dealing with new words or subject-specific words.

> Vygotsky coined the term *'zone of proximal development'* (ZPD) to refer to the presentation of a task that is just beyond the child's unaided ability, but not so difficult that they cannot succeed with adult support. The support is usually in the form of structured questions that guide attention to and reflection about the problem, and develop thinking.

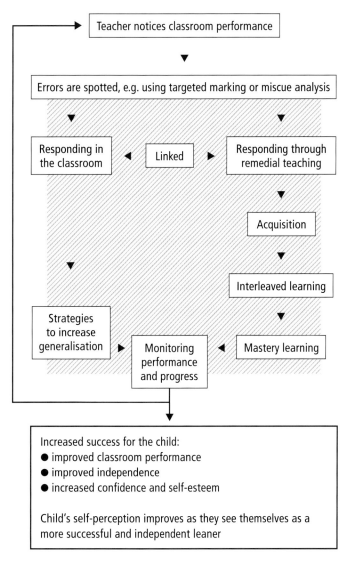

The flowchart contains:

Teacher notices classroom performance

Errors are spotted, e.g. using targeted marking or miscue analysis

Responding in the classroom ◄ Linked ► Responding through remedial teaching

Acquisition

Interleaved learning

Strategies to increase generalisation ► Monitoring performance and progress ◄ Mastery learning

Increased success for the child:
● improved classroom performance
● improved independence
● increased confidence and self-esteem

Child's self-perception improves as they see themselves as a more successful and independent leaner

IEPs and beyond SMART targets

Most schools have developed their own format for setting out Individual Education Plans or they make use of a standard format produced by their LEA. The model in the Code of Practice uses the IEP to guide remedial teaching. An example format is shown on page 30.

There is a wide variety of practice when using IEPs. I have seen IEPs from some schools that include over 20 targets and have been set up in September to run through the school year. It is unlikely that the teacher can deal with so many targets, especially as there will be more than one pupil in the class needing an IEP.

Sometimes targets are woolly and are couched in terms that are unrealistic, e.g. '*the pupil's reading age will increase by 6 months in the next 4 weeks*'. Sometimes targets on the IEP reflect teaching targets for the curriculum being presented to the class. This is not necessary – IEPs should only include targets that are *different* and *additional*.

Good practice requires some prioritisation. The IEP is usually devised for a short period of time and has 3 or 4 short-term targets that are:

- **S**pecific
- **M**easurable
- **A**ttainable
- **R**elevant
- **T**ime limited

Ideally, the IEP should be set up with parents involved as equal partners. The pupil should also be able to give their views and have these included in the planning.

The strategies should involve highly structured programmes that are carried out frequently. They should have an emphasis on success, work to develop mastery learning and include some element of interleaved learning. Interleaved learning allows some previously learnt material to be included when learning new material and has two advantages:

- it increases the child's confidence because the material is familiar and they succeed easily, and
- it refreshes learning after a period when the skill or material has not been practised. This deals with the problem of children appearing to forget a skill that they had previously mastered. Relearning is usually quicker than the original learning and this suggests that something of the original memory may remain.

How the teaching is to be resourced is an important issue. There are several questions to be answered:

- **What** is to be used? What materials or learning packages are needed?
- **Who** is going to carry out the intervention?
- **When** is the remedial work going to be done?
- **How long** is going to be spent during each session on this strategy?
- **How often** is the strategy going to be used?

Monitoring of learning is important. It allows us to know whether the strategy chosen is effective or not. It also provides useful information about when a target has been reached and it is time to move on. The monitoring does not need to be carried out every time learning takes place but it should be built into the programme at regular intervals. Good monitoring allows the rate of progress to be gauged and this can help future planning.

Exit criteria simply state the level to which the skill has to be mastered before the target is considered to have been met. This means that either a new target can be set or the time for remedial teaching can be divided amongst the remaining targets to provide a more focused intervention.

In-class support

The second aspect of supporting children with dyslexia requires teachers to plan to go beyond the IEP. The two main features to include are:

- opportunities for generalisation from remedial teaching to classroom work, and
- classroom support strategies to be used.

The main difficulty is that the support strategies need to be communicated, in an efficient way, to all those people who will teach the child. In a secondary school, this may be twelve or fifteen different teachers. Arrangements also need to be in place for days when the usual teacher is absent or out on a training course.

Generalisation is helped with good liaison between the teacher and adults working with the child on remedial programmes (either on a withdrawal basis, small group basis or in teaching specific strategies in the classroom by working alongside the child).

The support strategies used in class can be drawn from the examples given in this book. They could also include a listing of useful aids, software and classroom support packages. As with the IEP, this sheet should only list those strategies that are not in common use in the classroom. As teachers become more familiar with the strategies that can be used to support dyslexic children in their classroom, the number of strategies needing to be recorded will be reduced.

The Classroom Support Plan on page 31 gives a possible format for sharing this information and as an aide memoir for planning lessons. Ideally, it would be photocopied onto the back of the IEP. Most importantly, it is a working document to support the child in the classroom and as such should be referred to by the teacher during every lesson.

The classroom support plan will probably be longer term than the IEP. However, like the IEP, it will need to be reviewed. Some strategies selected for the pupil may turn out to be ineffective; others may become redundant as the child makes progress.

Individual Education Plan

Pupil name

Concern that has been prioritised

Start date   End date

Target	Strategies	Resources	Monitoring arrangements	Exit criteria

Classroom Support Plan		
Pupil name	Start date	End date
Opportunities for generalisation		
Useful information that the class teacher or subject teacher can collect to support specialist teaching		
Technological aids		
Classroom strategies		

The following example shows how the IEP and Classroom Support Plan might be used together. This is not intended to be a perfect example, it is given to model how the forms could be used.

Harry is an eight year old. His teacher thinks that he is 'quite bright' and cites him being able to answer questions in class discussions and having a good memory for facts. He can easily alliterate and rime and seems to have a good phonological awareness – so long as no print is involved. In his reading, he often confuses similar looking letters. A piece of recent writing gives an idea of his spelling – 'i ga naw on a dus' [I go home on a bus]. At first these spellings appear bizarre. However, a closer look shows that he:

● confuses similar looking letters by orientation (b/d, h/n, w/m),
● confuses similar shaped letters (a/o), and
● has not learnt the orthographic rule for adding 'e' to make a long vowel sound (magic e rule).

Harry does not have a Statement and is currently supported at School Action Plus. His parents are very supportive, but busy and can only afford a few minutes each day to work with him. His mum is quite anxious that Harry 'plays her up' when she tries to work with him on reading and spelling.

A number of possibilities exist for choosing targets for Harry:

● improving discrimination between similar looking letters when reading,
● improving discrimination between similar looking letters when writing,
● learning specific words to improve reading and spelling (e.g. bus, home),
● working on the 'magic e rule',
● learning rules to help with all long vowel sounds,
● learning more general orthographic rules, and
● develop proof reading skills involving looking up words in a personal dictionary or word list.

These would be discussed between his teacher and parents at a planning meeting and a choice made. Once targets have been selected, materials are considered and strategies chosen. Monitoring is considered and exit criteria determined. The work of teaching Harry is then divided up.

The difficulty that Harry has in recording his ideas independently in class work is recognised and his teacher considers ways that might support him in class. The combined plan is shown on the next two pages.

Individual Education Plan

Pupil name   *Harry*

Concern that has been prioritised

Harry confuses similar looking letters when reading and spelling

Start date   *1 Sep 02*   End date   *18 Oct 02*

Target	Strategies	Resources	Monitoring arrangements	Exit criteria
Be able to discriminate between b/d when writing	Daily practice of 10 words chosen from list for quick spelling test with parents at home (M, T, W), adult helper during registration (Th, F)	Spelling lists of phonically regular words containing b/d	Score from Friday spelling tests	10 out of 10 on two successive weeks
Be able to discriminate between b/d/ p/q and between h/n when reading	Daily practice of letter recognition with teaching assistant after break each afternoon	Precision teaching charts with randomly presented target letters produced on computer and printed on sheets. Stop watch for timing one minute for fluency training	Weekly probe sheets to measure number of letters correctly identified in one minute	30 letters identified correctly in one minute on two successive probe sheets
Successfully identify b/d in class reading book	Peer tutoring with instruction to look for 'b' and 'd', daily before lunch	More competent peer trained to engage in peer tutoring and instructed in searching for 'b' and 'd'	Weekly check by teaching assistant and recorded to show percentage of letters identified	85% accuracy in spotting b/d correctly

2

Classroom Support Plan

| Pupil name | Harry | Start date *1 Sep 02* End date *Dec 02* |

Opportunities for generalisation	Looking for b/d during literacy hour whole class reading, group reading and supported individual reading Targeted marking of writing to highlight b/d errors Teacher modelling choosing b/d in whole class teaching and teaching mnemonic using hands to make letters
Useful information that the class teacher or subject teacher can collect to support specialist teaching	Evidence from targeted marking to inform choice of b/d words for practice spellings at home
Technological aids	b/d visual mnemonic cue cards sellotaped to corner of desk Electronic spell checker to allow Harry to check some words for himself Tape recorder so that the teacher can record reading to support Harry during class work Tape recorder so that Harry can record some of his answers and ideas rather than writing them down
Classroom strategies	Sit near front so that teacher can easily provide support during reading or writing. Provide support 'in passing' Sit next to more competent peer (John) to support class reading and following worksheet instructions Being allowed to stick worksheets into book and writing short answers to questions directly onto sheet Cloze procedure for some writing Introducing Harry to the idea of the 'magic line' to encourage independent writing Personalised word list to copy words from during independent writing Key words put on board during class discussion about writing Key words for different curriculum areas displayed on walls, along with routine words such as days of the week

Differentiation

Children learn at different rates and this needs to be reflected in the approach taken by teachers and teaching assistants. The slower readers and spellers need more support while the faster readers and spellers need extending and pushing. This is referred to as differentiation within the classroom and can take many forms:

- *Differentiation by task* – different groups of children within the classroom are given different tasks linked to the teaching theme for the lesson.
- *Differentiation by outcome* – all of the children are given the same task but expected to vary in the quality, length or complexity of response. If the task is to record thoughts and discussions about a character in a book for example, some pupils may write several paragraphs of prose, others may make a list or a mind map, or sketch an illuminating scene from the book.
- *Differentiation by support* – all of the children get the same task and are expected to complete it to a similar standard but some children get more support than others. This support could include adding structure to the task (e.g. using writing frames) or could be adult support to complete some parts of the task. Group working allows children to support each other, e.g. a dyslexic child might be supported by a more competent reader who might in turn benefit from the scintillating array of ideas generated by the dyslexic child. Technological support can be used to enable a poor reader to access text more successfully or a poor writer to record ideas more independently. The next chapter contains ideas that teachers and parents can use to support their children.

The amount of support provided needs to be sufficient for the child to succeed but not so much so that it prevents the child from becoming an independent learner.

Learnt helplessness

Some pupils appear to over-rely on adult support, waiting until the teacher or assistant is working with them before attempting things well within their capability. They become dependent on being 'led by the nose' and this reduces their ability to learn and problem solve. This learnt helplessness is often associated with faulty beliefs such as, *'I must not be able to do it otherwise Miss would not be helping me. After all, she doesn't help anyone else!'*

In order to prevent this from happening it is necessary for the person supporting the child (teacher, teaching assistant, parent helper or parent) to consider a range of questions. This will allow effective support without encouraging dependency.

- Can I support a small group of children rather than an individual?

- Can I ask questions that prompt the children to think about strategies to use in order to solve the problem for themselves?
- How can I direct their attention to the important features of words when reading?
- How can I encourage them to make comparisons with words that they already know?
- Can I encourage them to take risks with learning, e.g. by guessing, praise their attempts, and show them where they have been successful (even if only partially)?
- Am I emotionally strong enough to refuse to help a child when I know that the task is well within their capability? Good monitoring of children's performance will allow me to remind the child of other occasions when they were able to do this task.
- How can I fade support as the child becomes more competent so that I am only providing the minimum level of help and encouraging the child to be independent? Can I leave the child longer before providing input, while at the same time expressing an expectation that they will successfully complete at least part of the task unaided?
- Can I make use of flow charts to take the child through routine procedures to increase the amount of time spent working independently? (Pictograms and teaching how to use the chart will decrease reliance on reading instructions or on adult support.)
- Can I make use of forward chaining? This is where the child starts off the first few steps of the problem and the adult helps them complete it. Gradually increasing the number of steps that the child is asked to do moves them towards greater independence.
- Can I make use of backwards chaining? In this case, the adult starts off the problem solving, leaving the child to complete the last few steps. As with forward chaining, gradually increasing the number of steps that the child is asked to do moves them towards greater independence.

Examples of chaining include encouraging children to try out spellings by getting them to write down as much of the word as they can remember and replace missing parts with dashes. In free writing, some teachers make use of a 'magic line'. This simply allows the child to write the words that they think they know and to use a *magic line* to represent the words that they do not know. This has the advantage of maintaining a flow in writing, supporting self-esteem and allowing the teacher to provide guided assistance after the initial draft.

Comparison with peers

Children do not like to be seen to be different from their peers. This is a problem that seems to become more acute as they reach adolescence. This has three major effects in school:

- The child compares himself to peers in terms of performance, particularly in literacy, and often finds himself wanting.

- The child does not want to be singled out in class by having a 'helper' sit with him.
- It can be difficult to make, and keep, friends.

In the first case, the child's self-esteem can be protected by having a positive class ethos in which each child is valued for what they can do. The teacher is able to show the child in a positive light in classroom activities and allow the child to demonstrate competence in some activities in front of their peers. The teacher tries hard to avoid depreciating remarks that carry the messages *'You are useless/worthless'*.

Parents and carers have a role to play in this as well. It is easy for parents' anxieties and worries about a lack of progress to be contained in unintentional messages to the child. This might be because the child sees the parent is always at school talking to the teacher and having 'worried conversations'. In some schools this is mitigated by having an open atmosphere where parents regularly meet with teachers at the end of the day. In this case the child could be given a task to do while the parent and teacher talk. Another strategy is to have a home-school book in which positive comments and concerns are exchanged. Not all parents find it easy to visit school to talk about their child, especially when 'unknown' specialists are involved (SENCo, specialist teacher, school nurse, educational psychologist, etc). Care should be taken to arrange such meetings at a time convenient to the parent, for example just after dropping their child at school or just before picking them up at the end of the day. Creating an informal and comfortable meeting place will put parents at ease and help to reassure them that their contribution is valued.

At home, parents should avoid talking to friends and relatives about the child's 'problems' while the child is listening. It is a natural response to a concern to want to talk it over with someone, but allowing the child to hear that his parents are worried, and giving him the impression that the 'whole world' knows about his failings, will not be very constructive.

The Code of Practice for Special Educational Needs places an emphasis on children being involved in their assessment and having a voice in reviews. This could be managed by having the child present as an equal partner in review meetings and having a discussion with a positive framing. This means that positive messages are used that focus on success – what can the child do today that he could not do last week?

In some schools, teachers use a 'dartboard' approach where each child sets one or two targets at a time. They write these on slips of paper with their name and pin them round the edge of the dartboard. They might be things such as:

- I want to read out loud in assembly by the end of term.
- I want to go up a level in maths by Christmas.

● I want to manage two weeks without detention.

As the children make progress, they move the targets closer to the bull's eye. Once they succeed, they write another target. This approach needs some negotiation with teachers and teaching assistants so that targets are realistic and achievable but it helps by encouraging the child to set goals and to monitor them. It also allows all of the children in the class to set their own personal targets and this is supportive because it is the 'normal thing' to do. A second advantage of this approach is that it can also alert the teacher to what is important to the child. In the first example given above, it had never occurred to the teacher that the child might want to read in assembly as he had always appeared to be disaffected and sardonic.

Summary

In designing a remedial programme and planning classroom support think about:

● Where is the child starting from? What can he do already?
● What are his strengths and weaknesses?
● Are there opportunities for over-learning and interleaved learning?
● How will learning be linked between the remedial programme and everyday classroom work in order to support generalisation?
● How does the remedial programme link to what the child needs in the classroom?
● How are links made between support staff and class or subject teachers?
● How can learning be 'fun'? For example, is there a variety of activities to teach the same knowledge or skills in a range of different ways?
● Who will do what and when will they do it?
● What specialist materials are needed?

Classroom Settings and Supportive Strategies

The classroom environment

John is writing a story. He wants to use a word that he is not sure about. He starts to look around the classroom where his teacher has placed 'key words' on almost every available surface. They appear on cupboards identifying their contents. They are hung on the wall naming the days of the week, months and seasons. They are displayed on the topic board – giving the specialist vocabulary needed for this term.

John's experience is a good example of how a teacher can create a supportive classroom environment. In a primary school, clear labelling of objects with pictograms as well as word labels will help with:

- acquiring reading skills of basic words used regularly in class,
- providing a model to support writing of familiar everyday words, and
- allowing pupils to find things easily and independently.

In a secondary school, the classroom is more likely to be used for only one or two subjects and this means that subject specific key words can be used. For instance in a science laboratory diagrams of each piece of commonly used equipment can be labelled as a model for pupils to use when writing up lab reports.

Other things to think about are:

- access to different resources within the classroom
  - word banks
  - spelling aids
  - a computer
  - books of different reading ages covering the same content range

- different types of pens/pencils
- location of aids to support dictionary skills and counting
  - alphabet arcs or lines
  - number lines
  - multiplication squares
- aids to remembering common sequences
  - days of the week
  - months of the year

Children will still need to be encouraged to make use of the information around them and further support might be needed.

Adult support

A range of adults can provide support in the classroom but the responsibility for teaching or co-ordinating teaching lies with the class teacher.

Classes vary in size and the amount of adult support available varies. Some classes may have fewer than twenty pupils while others will be over thirty. Some classes will have only one teacher while others will have teaching assistants, parent helpers, and other volunteers.

Fortunately, very few children require one-to-one support all of the time. This means that a range of strategies can be used:

- The teacher can circulate around the class rather than remaining at a fixed workstation. This allows for frequent but short visits to ensure that the child is still coping with the reading or writing task. Short prompts can be given in passing and the child re-assured frequently.
- Direct support through assisted writing or acting as a scribe or a reader.
- Reading through written feedback with the child so that they are aware of the comments made by the teacher.
- Giving help with spelling words that they are unsure about.
- Repeating significant points of the lesson in different forms, e.g. providing structured verbal questions or additional discussion that allows the child to explore concepts at a different level.
- One-to-one discussion can provide different angles to get the same point across.
- Adult support might be needed for assessment in key subjects.
- Support can be used to provide regular reinforcement of new skills/ knowledge or skills taught in remedial work to encourage generalisation.

Peer support

A shortage of adult time does not mean that children cannot be supported in class. A more competent peer can sometimes be used to support a weaker child. This could include:

- Paired reading
- Acting as a reader

- Acting as a scribe
- Acting as a checker, e.g. proof reading the child's script and identifying three spelling errors, or a 'critical friend'
- As a 'tester' for spellings, etc.

With a positive and supportive ethos operating in the classroom, the more competent child can act as a role model for the dyslexic child in order to support literacy development. Care needs to be taken in the choice of 'pairings' for this purpose however, and some sort of preparation or training for the 'peer tutor' is advisable. Consideration should be given by the 'peer tutor' to having a positive approach at all times, and knowing how to help without 'doing it for him'.

Often, the dyslexic child will be able to do some things better than the child supporting him with reading, and this means that the support is able to flow in both directions. Care should be taken that the arrangement does not in any way disadvantage the more able pupil, as outlined in this parent's views:

"Richard was always good at science, top of the class. But he was paired up with a dyslexic boy and always had to help him. I felt that he should have been doing extension work, more challenging stuff to keep him interested and stretch him. But he was always saddled with John, and often ended up spending his break times helping him to finish off his work."

Seating

Should the teacher sit all children with special needs on one table so that she can spend more time with them as a group? On face value this seems to have clear advantages, however, it can mean that dyslexic children are not suitably challenged – they need support with literacy while being given content that is demanding. The danger of having all children with SEN on one table is that opportunities for presenting more demanding work are lost.

The alternative is to sit children in mixed ability groupings. This has the advantage of providing more appropriate social mixes and allowing the dyslexic child to access complex work with peers. If the child is sitting with other children of the same intellectual ability then they can participate in discussions at an appropriate level. This may also be protective of self-esteem for a bright dyslexic child.

The disadvantage is that the teacher has to move about more in order to provide support for reading and writing.

The following strategies might help:

- Sit the child near to the teacher's table to allow easy access to adult support and to allow the teacher to monitor progress.
- Sit the child near to, and facing the board to help with:
  - copying by reducing the time taken from looking at the target

information and writing it down (helps reduce working memory demands).

- providing good literacy models from the class teacher.
- providing a clear focus for board-based explanations.

● Position the child near to/in clear sight of displayed flow diagrams and key words to support instruction-following and extended writing.

If the child is left handed, consideration will need to be given about whom the child sits next to and on which side. It is easy for left- and right-handed children to be placed next to each other so that they tend to crowd each other out when writing. (Left-handers need to have extra 'elbow room' on their left side, so should always sit to the left of a right-handed classmate.) The teacher will need to ensure that there is sufficient room for children to sit with correct posture and balance when writing and have sufficient space to place reference materials.

Coloured overlays

Coloured overlays can help some dyslexic children and it is always worth keeping some in the classroom. These are clear sheets of plastic, like OHP transparencies, in a range of colours. They work by changing the background colour of the text and reducing the high contrast between print and paper. When these are placed over the text, some pupils say *'the words have stopped jumping about!'*. Research indicates that many students read more quickly and effectively using the overlays.

Access to text on the computer

If black print on a white background is proving a problem, change the colours on the word processor. Right click on an empty area on the desktop. This will bring up a menu; click on *Properties* to open up the *Display Properties* window. Click on the *Appearance* tab and in the *Item* box, choose *Window*. You can now choose different colours for text and background. Black text on a grey background is less painful to the eyes than the standard white 'paper' but each user may have different preferences. It is quick and easy to change colours.

What else can be provided?

There is a range of devices that might help. One example is the Visual Tracking Magnifier (VTM), designed by Ian Jordan and produced by Combined Optical industries, which won a Millennium Award. It is a magnifying glass with a clear window across the centre for viewing groups of words and a patterned area above and below to block out interference from surrounding text.

"The VTM is easily tracked across a page and works by eliminating the pattern glare that confuses visual dyslexics. It also increases spatial differences between lines.

It consists of a specially designed pattern printed onto a bright field magnifying glass. A central clear rotatable band magnifies words so that they can be easily broken into their component parts.

Research
Arnold Wilkins has undertaken a controlled experiment using a Colorimeter to investigate the effects of coloured lenses and overlays on dyslexia. The Colorimeter allows a child to select the colour that they find most useful in reducing any effects of glare. This can be used as a coloured overlay or built into a pair of coloured glasses. Wilkins showed that coloured overlays increase the rate of reading and reduce visual stress, even in children with no known deficit within the school system.
Using a Rate of Reading test, in which 15 common words are presented in random order, children who chose to use a coloured overlay read faster. This test is difficult to see, but the words themselves are simple, making it easy to read and thus providing a good measure of any visual problems. More than 50% of the children reported improved perception with coloured filters, and 47% chose the same colour in response to different assessment methods and examiners. Their improvement in reading fluency persisted at retest.
http://www.essex.ac.uk/ psychology/overlays/

Visit Ian Jordan's website: www.visualdyslexia.com

Asfedic tuning
A company called Tintavision has been trialling 'asfedic tuning' with a small number of schools. This is a process designed to rapidly improve a person's reading speed, accuracy and stamina by finding the most appropriate filter. Specialist software is used to find the exact shade of filter from some 16 million choices, to maximise the rate of reading and reading stamina. The company provides a filter and arranges return visits where the filters will be changed after further testing. In time, many pupils have reached a stage where they can read efficiently without filters of any kind as their eyes are tuned to deal with the text they meet in day to day life.
Tel: 01778 349 233;
Fax: 01778 345 599;
www.tintavision.com

The device should assist nearly all early readers struggling with the mechanics of reading and a proportion of older pupils with difficulties.

The VTM is designed to reduce pattern glare without the use of tints. It aids fixation and may promote 'good' saccadal eye movement. Flicker is also reduced… It could be used in conjunction with other treatments, tinted spectacles for example."
Jordan, I., *Visual Dyslexia A guide for parents and teachers* (Desktop Publications, 2000)

Where pupils are benefiting from using overlays, it might be worth considering the Optim-Eyes™ Task Lamp, also produced by Ian Jordan. Overlays are useful for reading but may not help the pupil who needs to compose and review what he has written.

"The Optim-Eyes™ lamp is colour selectable, allowing colours to be mixed to create the optimum lighting to suit each user. The lamp can be used in addition to specifically prescribed tinted spectacles to achieve optimum results. The colour selection can be operated wither individually or together so that it is possible to select single primary colours or combine them to give different hues and luminance that can be used for both reading and writing."
Jordan, I., *Visual Dyslexia Signs, Symptoms and Assessment* (Desktop Publications, 2002)

Supportive strategies

How can pupils with reading and spelling difficulties be supported in mainstream classrooms and included in the curriculum? Ofsted (1999) surveyed over 50 schools and found that pupils' responses were better when teachers understood the difficulties of the children and made allowances for this in the work presented and in their teaching style. Where the quality of teaching was unsatisfactory it was because the teachers had unrealistic expectations of what the children could read and how much of their understanding they could demonstrate in writing. When teachers received training and support they were better able to take difficulties into account and plan appropriately for the pupils. This echoes a theme from the Code of Practice for SEN – teachers notice children's difficulties and respond by adjusting their teaching appropriately.

There are many things that teachers can do for pupils in every lesson to support literacy. Cooper and McIntyre (1993) found a number of commonalities between pupil perceptions and teacher perceptions of effective classroom practice. Ofsted (1999) found similar effective practices being used with children who did not have direct support through a Statement of SEN. Some of these are relevant to supporting pupils with reading and writing difficulties:

● teacher discussions (recapping from previous lessons; story telling; leading class discussions; teacher explanations; teacher exposition of ideas)

- use of the board (notes and diagrams as an aide memoir)
- use of pictures and other visual stimuli (including video material)

In this chapter we are going to present a range of ways of responding to children's needs. Not all of the strategies will be needed with all children, but there are sufficient ideas to allow a graduated response.

Supporting classroom reading

Teachers can support children with literacy difficulties by carefully selecting books for them and by thinking about how text is used when preparing worksheets. Text can be differentiated in a number of ways:

Language structure

Think about the language structure used in the books, worksheets, computer programs and board work used with the child. Is it at a level that they can cope with? Many of the indices for measuring reading ages of text consider sentence length, syllable counts and word familiarity. This is because:

- long sentences are harder to read than short ones. More demand is made on the memory to hold onto the ideas contained in the sentence. This means that less use can be made of sentence context to predict what the next words will be.
- high frequency words are encountered more often in reading and are more likely to be in the child's vocabulary.
- longer words place more demands on auditory memory for beginner readers than short words. Polysyllabic words make more demands on working memory for children who have learnt to chunk letters into sound groups.
- active verbs are easier to understand than passive verbs. Whether a verb is active or passive depends on how it is used in the sentence. For example, both of the following sentences mean the same but the first one is easier to read and understand:
  - The cat chased the dog. (Active)
  - The dog was chased by the cat. (Passive)

Emotional impact

Tightly-packed text can be overwhelming to a child who is struggling with reading. They see a lot of words on the page and somehow they have to make sense of what is being said. This can be so off-putting that the child tries to avoid the task. The equivalent experience for an adult would be a bit like reading a very academic, theoretical book on dyslexia! The following suggestions will help to make it easier (and some have been employed in thinking about this book):

- *Small blocks of text with spaces clearly defined.* This includes the use of:
  - Paragraphs – white space is important. As well as separating ideas, it gives emotional reassurance – the page becomes a set

of little chunks to be read.

- Boxes and frames – separate out ideas or functions within the text. For example, have instructions in one box and an explanation in another.
- Colour-coding of text – can make it easier for the teacher or parent to guide the child, *'just read the blue bit'*.
- Use of bullet points and lists rather than continuous prose – helps present ideas quickly without wasting time decoding text that carries no information other than the niceties of the English language.
- Use of diagrams and pictures – breaks up the text. These also convey important visual information that can help children to quickly understand the relationships between ideas and how these relate to the text. Pictures need to be chosen carefully so that they do not distract. They can be humorous, and may be the first thing that the child looks at – they act to draw the child into the book or worksheet.

- *Larger text.* This can give the child the feeling of moving swiftly through a page or book.
- *The look of the book.* Many dyslexic children are aware of their difficulties with reading and believe that other children will think they are stupid if they cannot read the same books as the rest of the class. This is made worse if they are reading books intended for younger pupils, especially if they are in a junior class reading an infant book. Teachers can make use of 'parallel readers' – books not used in school for the majority of readers but saved for those who need extra practice at every stage.

Aaron is a year 5 pupil whom I observed in class. The pupils were spending ten minutes quietly reading while the teacher took the register and got materials ready for a science lesson.

Aaron had taken out a thick tome – *Harry Potter*. Other children on the table were reading similar books and he desperately wanted to read it. The book was far too difficult for Aaron and he spent most of the time looking around the classroom, flicking backwards and forwards through the pages and fiddling with his pencils.

His teacher noticed and asked him to take out his 'reading book'. Instead of a thick paperback book like the other children had, out came a thin hardback from the school's reading scheme. The book is just at a level that Aaron can read – but he doesn't want to. It is not what the other children are reading about. How many nine- year-olds want to read a story written for six-year-olds? Aaron lay it on his table and volunteered to help give out equipment.

Competency and reading

The demands of the text need to be matched to the abilities of the child. The teacher reflects on whether or not the child can read 90% of a sample of the text without direct support. At this level, the child will encounter two words out of every twenty that are 'difficult'. He will be able to decode sufficient information to make use of sentence meaning and word attack skills to make a reasonable guess at the word. This is how competent readers become better readers.

Checking text readability

The Five Finger test
This is a quick way to check the suitability of a book for a child. It is not foolproof, but is easy enough for children to learn themselves and employ when choosing a book from the library, class reading box or bookshop. It works with 'chapter books' where there are more than just a couple of sentences on a page. Choose a page in the middle of the book, ask the child to read the text out loud. Each time he comes across a word that he cannot read, tell him the word and count the word with a finger. If you run out of fingers before you reach the end of the page then the text is probably too hard.

Use a word-processor to check reading ages
You could scan or type the text into a word processor and then use the in-built readability statistics to tell you the reading age. In Word, go to the *Tools* menu, click *Options*, then click the *Spelling and Grammar* tab. Select the *Check grammar with spelling* check box. Select *Show the readability statistics* check box, then click *OK*. Click *Spelling and Grammar* on the *Standard toolbar*. When Word finishes checking spelling and grammar, it displays information about readability of the text.

The **Flesch-Kincaid Grade Level** is reported by Microsoft Word. The number given is the average reading ability for pupils in the school year in the US education system. Adding 5 to the number produces a reading age. It can be calculated by hand using the following steps:

1. Count the number of words in the sample.
2. Count how many sentences are in the sample.
3. Find the average sentence length by dividing the number of words by the number of sentences.
4. Now multiply this number by 0.39.
5. Count the number of syllables in the sample.
6. Divide the number of syllables by the number of words.
7. Multiply this number by 11.8.
8. Add your answer from step 4 to your answer from step 7, then subtract 15.59 to get the grade level.
9. Add 5 to get the reading age.

There are many ways of calculating reading ages. A slightly simpler way than the previous example is the **Fog Index**. This tends to work better with older pupils:

1. Open the book randomly at three different places and count 100 words in each place to give three samples.
2. Count how many sentences there are in each sample. For incomplete sentences, estimate how much of the remaining sentence in each sample is included in the sample (to the nearest tenth).
3. Work out the average sentence length by dividing 300 by the total number of sentences in the three samples.
4. Count how many words have three or more syllables in the three samples. Divide this number by three (to give an average).
5. Add together your answers from step 3 and step 4.
6. Multiply this by 0.4 to get the grade level.
7. Add 5 to get the reading age.

Sources of suitable readers
A much easier way is to look at publishers' websites to see suggested age ranges of different books. Look out for 'High interest, low reading ages'. These are designed to motivate older readers while still having a low reading age.

The Dyslexia Institute also lists hundreds of books suitable for dyslexic readers. Tel: 01784 463 851 or email: info@dyslexia-inst.org.uk

A graded list of reading books is available from the National Association for Special Educational Needs. Tel: 01827 311 500 or email: welcome@nasen.org.uk

Exposure to print for a child who has grasped the basics means that he can learn more about reading and increase his sight vocabulary, reading fluency and verbal repertoire through reading. The difficulty for the teacher of a dyslexic child is providing text at a reading level that allows this level of accuracy, while also being meaningful to the lesson or to the child. There are a number of reading schemes available that have high interest levels but low reading ages for older children with reading difficulties.

Improving worksheet layout to support reading

All of the principles that apply to selecting books for children also apply to worksheet design. When designing a worksheet, the teacher can think about:

- breaking up large chunks of text. Have plenty of sub-headings as signposts and markers. You can support organisational difficulties if questions related to the text are included in the same box, along with a space to write the answer. In comprehension exercises, this will also help children with working memory deficits by reducing the attentional capacity demands needed to remember the location of the text they were reading as they ponder the answer to the question asked. This will reduce the need to re-read the text from the beginning if the child suddenly loses their place. For example, instead of having three paragraphs of text and then six questions, split the text into paragraphs, with two questions placed under each. Each block can then be placed in a box to emphasise the structure of the information. Reading is supported because the child does not need to re-read the whole of the text in order to find the answers.

Text Text Text Text Text Text Text Text Text Text Text Text Text Text Text Text Text Text Text Text Text Text Text Text Text Text Text Text Text Text Text Text Text Text Text Text Text Text Text Text Question 1 Question 2 Question 3 Question 4 Question 5 Question 6	Text Text Text Text Text Text Text Text Text Text Text Text Text Text Question 1 Question 2
	Text Text Text Text Text Text Text Text Text Text Text Question 3 Question 4
	Text Text Text Text Text Text Text Text Text Text Text Text Text Text Text Question 5 Question 6

- supporting text with visual cues, e.g. pictures, diagrams, flow charts.
- making sure that sheets are typed rather than handwritten. This is to provide a consistent model of print for the child to recognise.

Choose a font that is clear and easy to read. The most dyslexia-friendly are generally thought to be Arial, Sassoon and **Comic Sans**.

- selecting a point size that is appropriate to the child. Use 12 or 14 point so that the pupil does not have to strain to read the words. Small text requires both eyes to scan and focus on a small area. Younger children find this difficult, as they have not yet developed ocular stability. In some older children, a lack of ocular stability makes the letters on the page appear to move. Enlarging the text provides a bigger target for both eyes to focus on.

- avoiding justified margins. Some pupils have major problems with 'channelling' – they are more aware of the spaces between the words than the words themselves. Often textbooks and handouts have justified margins to make the page look neat. These work by using irregular spacing between words so there is a tidy right-hand margin. Where pupils have problems with tracking or maintaining a smooth flow across a line of text, they are likely to find such pages harder to read.

Some pupils have major problems with 'channelling' – they are more aware of the spaces between the words, than the words themselves. Textbooks and handouts frequently have justified margins to make the page look neat. These work by using irregular spacing between words, so there is a tidy right-hand margin. Where pupils have significant problems with tracking, or maintaining a smooth flow across a line of text, they are likely to find such pages harder to read.

Note the irregular spacing between words.

Some pupils have major problems with 'channelling' – they are more aware of the spaces between the words, than the words themselves. Textbooks and handouts frequently have justified margins to make the page look neat. These work by using irregular spacing between words, so there is a tidy right-hand margin. Where pupils have significant problems with tracking, or maintaining a smooth flow across a line of text, they are likely to find such pages harder to read.

Worksheets that give instructions

If the worksheet is giving instructions for practical work, try to put each new instruction on a new line. Number the instructions to support the child's organisation and memory. If possible support with pictures. See example on page 49.

Growing plants

This week

You will need: a ruler, 2 plants about the same size, 2 labels.

1. Write 'Dark' on one label.
2. Measure one of the plants with a ruler.
3. Write the height of the plant in the table.
4. Put the label onto the pot.
5. Put the plant in a dark cupboard.
6. Write 'Light' on the other label.
7. Measure the other plant with a ruler.
8. Write the height into the table.
9. Put the label onto the pot.
10. Put the plant on the windowsill.
11. Leave for one week (make sure they both have enough water).

	Plant in **DARK** place	Plant in **LIGHT** place
Height at start		
Height after one week		

Next week

1. Measure each plant again.
2. Put the new heights into the table.

How much has each one grown?

Teacher strategies when working with the whole class

- Start by directing pupils' attention to the text to be read by holding the book up to the class and identifying the area to be read:
  - point at the target text,
  - identify the colour of text box,
  - state the paragraph number, and
  - use other cues, e.g. "under the picture", "on the left page, half-way down", "just before the questions".
- Pre-read the text with the class so that the child feels more confident when approaching independent reading. This also allows the child to make use of memory strategies to reduce the need to rely on fluent reading.
- Carry out whole class discussion of the text prior to individual work.
- Use different coloured chalk or white board markers with each line of writing to be copied from the board, to help the child scan and re-locate the next target word to be written. If the child has difficulty remembering where they were up to, they may find it easier to remember that they were on the green line. Take care to check for contrast in different parts of the room and at different times of day – blue chalk on a blackboard looks fine until the sun shines on it! Alternatively, number each line of text.

Other strategies

- An adult can pre-read text with the pupil prior to use in the lesson so that the difficult bits are identified and dealt with. This then improves confidence for independent reading during the actual lesson. Parents can be involved in this type of support if there is good liaison between home and school. Parents could read with their child using a paired reading approach or an apprenticeship model approach (see page 91).
- The child can have direct support in class through assisted reading by the teacher, teaching assistant or a more competent peer.
- A computerised script reader can be used in class. This consists of special software to read text files from the computer. Some versions of this are available free from the Internet. The latest version of Microsoft Word includes a speech option that will enable the computer to read highlighted text. This could be used to read back the child's work or work prepared by the teacher. When linked with a scanner and used with Optical Character Recognition (OCR) software, it is possible to scan any text and have the computer read it out to the child. Although this software is good and getting better, it does have a number of disadvantages.
  - It needs a relatively fast machine to work on and older machines may not cope with the demands, or may read too slowly.
  - The voice is mechanical and often has an American accent.
  - Syllables are not emphasised naturally.
  - Initials, acronyms and compound words are incorrectly pronounced.

Obtaining text to speech software
The following websites have versions of software available for converting text to speech:

www.ReadPlease.com
ReadPlease is a free download that works fine with highlighted text

www.elantts.com
Provides a demo version

www.infovox.se/demo.htm
Provides a demo version

www.loriens.com
A company that writes software specifically for dyslexics and has a demo version to try

These problems are not insurmountable, but require some time in training the child to use the software. The use of headphones is recommended to reduce distractions to the rest of the class, and to minimise interference from background noise.

- A ruler can be used to help with tracking in reading. A clear plastic ruler can be placed under the target text and this allows the child to see the next words on the line. It also allows the child to gauge how much of the page is left to read. A *linetracker* (LDA) does a similar job – possibly with more 'street cred'.

- A cardboard mask can be made that exposes one or two words at a time. This is useful if the child continues to have difficulty looking at the target word(s). A more sophisticated aid is the Jordan Visual Tracker Magnifier – a small lens that is placed over the target word to enlarge it and develop eye-tracking skills (see page 42).

- A photocopier can be used to enlarge text, which aids binocular control. A bigger target on the page helps children who say that they experience the words moving on the page. An A4 magnifier could be used instead – but check quality carefully as the prismatic effect can cause interference patterns that spoil the image and make reading more difficult.

- Some children can be helped when writing is on coloured paper. It might be worth experimenting to see if a particular shade or colour helps improve reading.

- Coloured overlays can also be used to help reduce apparent movement of letters. The *Irlen Test* is a test for scotopic sensitivity that can help identify which colour filter is best. Some ophthalmologists will do this test and will prescribe coloured lenses. The *Wilkins Rate of Reading Test* can be used to explore the type of overlay that works best for children in years 4 to 6 (see page 42).

- A taped commentary of the class text being read can be provided so that the child can re-wind and re-listen to the text, e.g. during comprehension exercises.

- The child can record his own voice to help with reading and to use with word cards to support reading development (e.g. with the Language Master system).

Strategies to help the child understand the purpose of reading and writing come from a simple mnemonic – the PQRS strategy for reading (Preview, Question, Read, Summarise):

- **Preview** – look over the text to see if there are clues as to what it is about. Picture clues, headings, boxes, etc give a quick idea. With more competent readers this is developed into scanning and skimming skills.

- **Raise questions** to be answered. What do we want to find out? This might be very pertinent in looking for specific information from a textbook. With a story we might want to know what happens to the main character.

- **Read** the text, expectations will already have been set up regarding what the text is about and this will help with predictive processing of which words might be coming next.

The Language Master system is available from Drake Educational.
Tel: 029 2056 0333
www.drakegroup.co.uk

- **Summarise** – briefly say what the text was about. What are the answers to the questions that were raised? If it is a story, then use this time to set up expectations for the next reading session – what might happen next?

There are also specific skills needed to deal with challenging text:

- **Word-segmentation** – how can I break this word down? Are there any smaller words in it that I recognise? Are there groups of letters that I have seen before, e.g. 'ing', 'ed'?
- **Syntactic checking** – does the structure of the sentence, as I have read it, make sense?
- **Semantic checking** – does the meaning of the sentence, as I have read it, make sense?

Supporting writing

How well should children be able to record information in writing? There is an expectation that all children should reach the 'average' level, as measured by SATs, but achievement in writing continues to lag behind that in reading. There is also a gender gap, with boys consistently doing less well than girls.

Key Stage and expected standard	Girls	Boys
KS1 standard 2	90%	82%
KS2 standard 4	68%	52%

Table 3: Gender difference in writing measured by SATs (Ofsted, 2002)

Many children will not be able to write as well as expected of 'average' pupils, and will need supporting in class: this is particularly relevant to dyslexic pupils. Writing is a very complex process for anyone – even practised adults. This applies particularly to the production of a piece of creative or persuasive text. Preparation for this is all-important – the opportunity to think and talk about ideas, plan a sequence and research any unfamiliar spellings. The task of putting pen to paper is much more achievable when the child knows what he wants to 'say'. This sort of preparation can be done in a group but will be most effective when led by a teacher or teaching assistant.

- Ask the pupils to answer only half of the questions on a comprehension exercise – all the odd numbers/all the even numbers/the first three and last three. Remember that the questions are likely to be gradated in difficulty so choose alternate questions in order to give the child a chance to think about the harder concepts as well as the easy ones.
- Have models of language on the walls and cupboards of the classroom.
- Provide common spelling lists of words used in each topic or have these specially prepared on word cards around the room.
- For some pupils this can be adapted to personal word banks. These can be in a format appropriate to the age and ability of the child –

Recording ideas and information in prose can move through a gradation:

- Voice recording, e.g. to a tape recorder.
- Dictation, e.g. to a peer or adult; to a computer with speech recognition software.
- Using copy-writing models, graduated from over-writing to under-writing.
- Copying.
- Using sentence makers – common words that the child needs are written on cards and the child assembles the sentence using the cards. The teacher checks the sentence and then the child copies the model into his book.
- Using disrupted information – instead of giving the child a block of text to copy, provide them with the sentences in a jumbled order. If the sentences are cut out before the lesson, they can re-assemble the order, checking the sequence with an adult or peer, and then copy them. This allows the child to apply some thought to their writing whilst being supported.
- Copying the bulk of the text but completing missed-out bits, e.g. cloze procedure, sentence completion. This can be graduated further, e.g. providing the answers for the child to choose from; having source text containing the answers; having only a blank space to fill.
- Writing independently, using key words provided by the teacher. Support independent writing by providing key words on the board, on cupboards in the classroom, on topic boards, in subject-specific dictionaries.
- Writing to dictation.
- Writing independently with help to organise ideas, e.g. using writing frames, writing independently after planning.
- Totally independent writing.

a little book, a tin, or envelope with words that they need to use or ask about frequently.

- In some classes, teachers have found it useful to have laminated sheets of high-frequency words in alphabetical order, which pupils can keep on their tables.
- Cue cards can help remind pupils of common mistakes that they make when writing.

Which

Witch

- If worksheets are used, then allow the child to write on the sheet, rather than copying into his book. This will help him to keep up with other children in the class by saving time re-reading and re-tracking the target text, and will help with slower writing speed and slower information processing speed.
- Reduce writing demands by teaching the child how to record information independently and effectively using mind maps and flow diagrams.
- Use sentence completion by providing most of the sentence as a model with space for the child to complete it. Gradation could include providing the answers in a jumble, which the child selects.
- Give the child a book to make into a personalised dictionary. They write in the words that they want to use but frequently get wrong, or do not know. Teach them how to use the dictionary.

- Provide an alphabet line or alphabet arc to assist with independent dictionary skills:

Aa Bb Cc Dd Ee Ff Gg Hh Ii Jj Kk Ll Mm Nn Oo Pp Qq Rr Ss Tt Uu Vv Ww Xx Yy Zz

- Some children become over-reliant on phonic strategies and spell words as they sound. Try providing them with the Aurally Coded English (ACE) dictionary. This allows the child to look up words as they sound and then to find the correct spelling.
- With more competent children, encourage proof-reading skills. Teach the children to check for spelling mistakes, grammar and then meaning. This is always easier to do with someone else's work than with your own. When you have written something, you know what it 'should' say! Train pupils to work with 'critical friends', where each checks the other's work.
- Encourage the use of an electronic spell-checker. These vary in complexity and price. The cheaper ones allow the child to type in the word as they think it should be typed and it then offers them several possibilities from which to choose. More expensive versions will provide definitions of the chosen word so that the child can check that they have the right meaning.
- Teach spelling as an integral part of every lesson.

There are several ways to record ideas and observations that involve very little writing, or none at all. The following were suggested by Year 6 children attending a centre for dyslexic pupils:

- Use a tape recorder
- Take photos with a digital camera and add text
- Use a video camera
- Make a recording using a computer and web cam
- Tell the teacher the answers
- Make a storyboard
- Make a poster
- Record information in a table

The use of technological aids is covered in Chapter 4.

Summary
There are many things that the teacher can do to make the classroom more 'dyslexia friendly'. This involves thinking about:

- the classroom environment,
- how human resource support is organised,
- how tasks can be supported and adjusted,
- how information is organised.

Using ICT to Help Dyslexic Learners

Modern technology can offer a great deal to all children but is especially valuable to dyslexic learners. Used wisely, it is highly motivating, time saving and enables pupils to produce work that looks extremely good. New hardware and software is being developed all the time, so it is worth exploring the market from time to time, to keep abreast of new developments. A company like REM is a good place to start as their catalogue contains products from all the major providers (www.r-e-m.co.uk). If it is possible to visit any of the educational exhibitions during the year, this is a good opportunity to see products demonstrated and ask for advice about specific pupils' needs (BETT, January, London; Education Show, March, Birmingham NEC; Special Needs North, May, Bolton; Special Needs London, November, London).

Laptops

The use of laptop computers has revolutionised school life for some dyslexic learners. They are able to transport the machines from class to class and, with practice, become very proficient at using them.

- Use a laptop computer with the spell checker enabled to provide instant feedback on spelling errors and to allow the child to select from a restricted range of possibilities. If the child cannot get their ideas down because the spell checker distracts them and stops their flow of thoughts, then turn it off and teach the child the habit of spell checking once the document is written.
- Dictation software allows the child to speak to the machine. This type of software is getting better, but the child will need a lot of training to use it effectively. Ideally it needs to be used with software that can read back what the machine thinks the child has said.

> Some software can work with existing word processor programs and helps with typing by predicting what word the child is going to enter. An example of this is *Penfriend*. *Penfriend* opens up a small window that floats over the main program window. As a few letters are typed a list appears in the floating window of words that the program thinks you are going to type. Each choice is listed along with the function key (F1 to F12) that you can press to complete the word. This makes typing much quicker for inexperienced typists. A useful feature is that it will speak out each letter as it is typed or the word if the function key is pressed. Once a full stop is reached the whole sentence is read out. If a block of text is highlighted it will read it all out for the pupil.
> Available from Penfriend Ltd of 30 South Oswald Road, Edinburgh EH9 2HG.

- Use a word processor to allow the child to produce neat copies of work for display, to take home or to stick in a class book.
- Training in keyboard skills is essential if the child is to keep up

with note taking. It should go beyond typing skills to include specialist keys and short cuts used with the software that the child needs.

● Mind mapping software enables the child to record ideas visually and without having to type everything out in prose. Software can be downloaded from the Internet on a 21–30 day trail basis (see box below).

● A computer can be used to record information in table form.

Several websites offer different ranges of commercial products – some have reduced rates for students or educational institutions:

● www.conceptdraw.com for *Concept Draw*.
● www.ygnius.com/site/0_home for *Ygnius*.
● www.mindjet.co.uk for *Mind manager 2002* and *Mind Manager Smart*.
● www.dyslexic.com for *Kidspiration* – an American program for children in the class age range Reception to Year 3. It offers simple mind mapping and a range of other visual thinking tools designed for use with emergent readers and writers. It will speak out words written on mind maps and pupils can record their own voices. Visual thoughts can be quickly transformed into a serial written document. Also available from iANSYST Ltd, Fen House, Fen Road, Cambridge CB4 1UN.

The power of word processing

Matthew, aged 15, is working towards GCSE History. He has enjoyed the lessons as the teacher makes sure there is lots of discussion around the source documents. He is particularly good at finding clues in photographs and cartoons, which other pupils miss. He can also interpret graphs quite well. He has problems however, in producing written answers that do justice to his historical understanding and knowledge.

He is working on the question: "Why did support for the Nazis increase in the period 1929–1933?"

Figure 2 on page 57 shows Matthew's hand written work. The deficiencies are obvious at a glance. It is untidy, the letters are not evenly formed, the spelling is weak and many common words such as 'people' are misspelt. The essay is also underdeveloped and disorganised. However, there are a number of good points too. It contains relevant material such as the growing fear of Communism, the dissatisfaction of the middle classes, the surge of prosperity and industry in the 1920s, and the loss of wealth after the Wall Street Crash. The answer needs reorganising, points need developing and some basic spellings need to be learnt, such as 'would', 'people', 'middle', 'factories', 'classes' and 'wealthy'. There is also some essential subject vocabulary such as 'Nazi', 'Communist' and 'reparations', which will never appear on a drill and practice spelling programme but which need to be mastered.

Figure 2

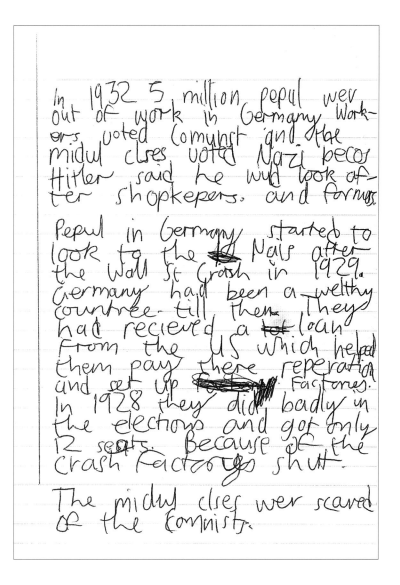

Spell checking

The use of a word processor makes the text legible and offers opportunities for different approaches to spelling. Matthew could use a spell checker by looking at each word that is underlined, right clicking the mouse and looking at alternatives, but there is a danger that he will accept

suggestions for corrections without learning anything. Some children see common words corrected so frequently that they learn the correct spelling subconsciously; others become aware, perhaps for the first time, that they have a particular problem with words and consciously register the correct spelling and make an effort the next time they want to use that word.

Track Changes

Another strategy is to use the *Track Changes* facility. This is on the *Tools* menu *(Tools, Track Changes, Highlight Changes)*. Be sure to click on the *Track Changes While Editing* box.

This facility records each change by crossing out text and substituting new words. When used in conjunction with the spell checker, it gives you a handy spelling list.

The only two items the spell checker did not cope with were 'there'/ 'their' and the word 'Nazis'. Matthew now has a set of spellings to work on and learn.

Using AutoCorrect and abbreviations

Some teachers and pupils may decide to speed up the writing process by using AutoCorrect to expand short forms of words. Many of us use abbreviations when we take notes – 'gov' for 'government', 'dev' for 'develop'. In this example, the pupil could put longer words on AutoCorrect. Alternatively, if Matthew is making extensive use of word processing for all subjects, he may start to use a wider range of abbreviations, e.g. 'wd' becomes 'would', 'shd' becomes 'should', to speed up his recording.

Some people see this as cheating, and worry that if the child is not laboriously writing out the words he will never learn to spell. However, writing is more than spelling and in this case, Matthew needs to write a history essay. The spelling is important but he needs to marshal ideas, produce a coherent and relevant account, be able to understand the significance of different events and justify his opinions. To this end, if the corrections on this work focus only on spelling then it becomes an English lesson and not a history task. No teacher or parent should ever lose sight of the fact that writing is much more than spelling, whatever the child's ability.

Developing ideas

There are many strategies that teachers use to raise the standard of pupils' work. Here are some of the most common:

- Have a list of questions for targeted reading and writing.
- Record questions on tape for poor readers.
- Get pupils to make a list of questions they want/need to find answers to. This leads to more purposeful reading and planning.
- Talk and create a spider diagram as a plan.
- Provide models of different writing (perhaps just a paragraph) so they can get the sound/tone/style in their heads.
- Keep good answers from previous years to read out to a class so they can see what they are aiming at.

Some teachers are using the *Insert Comment* facility on the *Insert* menu to develop digital marking.

This is where the teacher's marking appears on the screen. This is particularly good for GCSE coursework where many rewrites are needed before the pupil produces a piece of work that accurately reflects his ability. For pupils with poor visual tracking skills, it is difficult to look at their work on screen and then look down at a print out with hand written comments on it and then back to the right place on the screen to make changes.

With digital marking, the teacher's comments are legible and are on screen, close to the relevant piece of the essay.

Research skills

Pupils with poor literacy skills often have problems knowing what to put into an essay and may be tempted to copy out large chunks from a book. In the past, they were limited by how tired their hand became but with the digital age, pupils can download great chunks from the Internet and throw them into an essay. It requires no physical stamina and is the work of a moment.

In order to help pupils overcome this temptation, teachers need to teach them how to summarise and help them to develop skimming and scanning skills. The Internet is full of information but much of it may be irrelevant to the topic, biased or inaccurate. Pupils need to learn to be critical readers. Two strategies can help here.

Using the highlighter

Download a piece of text from the Internet and get pupils to use the highlighter tool to pick out the main points. As they run the tool over the words they get a yellow background. If they change their mind, run the highlighter over the words again and the colour disappears.

This extract is taken from a website and has been copied into Word so Matthew can read the text and identify relevant material for his essay.

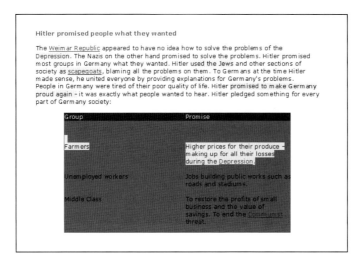

Making notes from key points

The Spike is a little known but very useful facility in Word that lets the user select bits of information and put it on the clipboard. It's a bit like *Cut* and *Paste* but it allows you to gather up lots of information from different parts of a document and then paste them all at once. It may be that you use the highlighter first to pick out the main points. Then run the cursor over each point in turn, pressing *Ctrl* and the *F3 key* to select the point. Keep going until you have all the points you want. The Spike will hold an almost indefinite amount of information. Then on a new document, press the *shift key, Ctrl* and the *F3 key* and it will paste all the material you have chosen.

> the Depression.
> used the Jews
> as scapegoats
> promised to make Germany proud again
> Farmers
> Higher prices for their produce – making up for all their
> losses during the Depression.

In newer versions of Word, you can select up to 24 pieces of information, which appear separately in a window at the side of your document. This gives users greater control over the order in which they want to use the information.

Now Matthew has a set of notes he can expand or incorporate into his essay. Again everything is in one place, on screen, and he is focusing on the writing task and not searching endlessly through books or notes or struggling with an index to find the page he wants. With the computer, he is in control and has an increasing range of strategies at his command in his quest to become an independent writer.

Summary

- Writing is more than spelling.
- With a word processor, you can produce legible text.
- Use a spell checker.
- Use the *Track Changes* facility in conjunction with the spell checker to produce a spelling list.
- Speed up the writing process by using AutoCorrect to expand short forms of words.
- Develop digital marking which is especially useful for pupils with poor visual tracking skills.
- Help develop skimming and scanning skills.
- Use the highlighter tool to pick out the main points in a text.
- Use the Spike or the clipboard to collect all the points you need from a text and then paste them as a set of notes or a plan.

4

Organisation and Planning Skills

General organisation

We often take it for granted that children will arrive on time to lessons with all of the things that they need. But this requires a high degree of skill, planning and organisation. Some dyslexic pupils develop a simple compensatory strategy – they carry everything with them for the whole week!

Parents can help by encouraging their child to develop good habits. They can:

- have a lesson and homework timetable visible at home and check it each night as their child arrives home from school (see page 64).
- establish a routine for homework – before/after tea, before school in the morning – and check that it has been completed.
- help their child to prioritise homework tasks – what needs doing for tomorrow, what can be left until the weekend (without creating a huge backlog!).
- help their child to get into the habit of preparing and packing his school bag ready for the next day.
- provide plastic wallets or envelope files for letters to and from school to increase the chances of messages being passed on correctly.
- provide a case for pencils, pens and rulers and have a good stock of spares at home to replace those lost or mislaid during the day.
- regularly check that the homework diary is being used and kept up to date.

Teachers can help by:

- having spare equipment that the pupil can borrow for the duration of the lesson if they have lost theirs. This should be done without fuss.
- prompting the child to take out necessary equipment and homework at the start of the lesson. Some teachers have this as an expectation for the whole class and encourage it through praise.
- writing important messages for parents in a home/school book. Some dyslexic children have poor memories and even if they remember there is something to tell their parents, they might not remember what it is.
- writing homework into the child's planner or asking a more competent peer to check that the child has written it down correctly, or providing a typed sheet.
- making it clear when work must be handed in.
- providing additional copies of timetables and school plans to increase the number of reference points for the child and take into account that they may not be organised enough to keep a

Sunday	Monday	Tuesday	Wednesday	Thursday	Friday	Saturday
	1	1	1	1	1	
	2	2	2	2	2	
	3	3	3	3	3	
	4	4	4	4	4	
	5	5	5	5	5	
	At home	At home	At home	At home	At home	
Pack swimming kit	Do homework for:	Do homework for:	Do homework for:	Do homework for:	Do homework for:	Make sure all sports kit and school uniform is washed
Check that all homework is done	Pack PE kit	Pack PE kit	Collect materials for D+T	Pack Karate kit	Pack PE kit	
Dinner money						
Bus fare/pass						

5

single copy with them at all times. Copies could be stuck into planners, put in their bedroom, on the fridge, on the form room notice board, in their locker, etc.

● regularly checking that the homework diary or planner is being used and kept up to date.

Extended writing

For a dyslexic child, the idea of attempting a large piece of independent writing can be daunting. Emotionally the task can seem impossible. Organisationally, it may result in an almost random presentation of ideas. Extended writing requires an element of planning and organisation. At the simplest level, this requires that the piece of work has a clear beginning, middle and end.

The teacher can support the child by providing the structure in the form of a writing frame. This breaks the overall task down into smaller sub-tasks, each with a clear indication of what is needed in each section. It also provides easy checkpoints for the teacher and pupil to review how the task is going.

Planning of extended writing can, and should, be taught. One method is to brainstorm, then use spider diagrams or mind maps to record ideas quickly. The ideas are then sequenced to produce the order in which they could be written. The next step is to write a rough draft for each idea. These are then written together with joining phrases (and signposts). Finally, the draft is read and adjusted to produce the final piece of work. This process can be modelled by the teacher and teaching assistant, with regular practice of each stage until the pupil is familiar with the process. An aide-memoire can be useful to keep pupils on task (see page 66).

Revision and coursework planning

Learning material for an examination requires a number of skills. Basic facts have to be memorised, processes have to be learnt and skills mastered. Previous examination papers can be used as a source of questions to allow the skills to be practised. The danger is that the child does not allow enough time to cover the entire syllabus or focuses too much on one area at the expense of the others.

Similar problems exist for coursework. Information has to be sought out, structured and then presented. Coursework usually has to be completed by set deadlines and for a whole range of subjects. At the start of a GCSE course these deadlines can seem a long way off and the child may do nothing during the early stages only to have a mad rush at the end of the course.

Parents and teachers can support the child by:

Writing essays and assignments

This piece of work is about: ....

In doing the work I need to: (find out/explore/decide/describe/consider/argue/discuss/comment on/evaluate/summarise)

....

....

The work should be about .... words/pages long.

The work should be hand written/word processed.

It must be handed in on ....

Before starting to write:

1. Do I understand what I have to do? (If not, ask your teacher, teaching assistant and/or a classmate.)
2. Have I got all the information I need? (Lesson notes, text book, library books, information from the Internet or from talking to other people.)
3. Make a list of your ideas/thoughts/facts/observations. Then make short notes on each one, using your own words to show your understanding. Leave plenty of space around your notes for extra thoughts, inserting 'better' words, etc. Put these points in a logical order.

When writing:

1. Introduce your work with a sentence or paragraph explaining what you are setting out to do.
2. Open each new paragraph with a clear explanation/statement/observation then use evidence or further information to 'flesh out' your ideas.
3. Finish with a closing paragraph that summarises what you have found out or what you think.

After writing:

1. Read through your work and check that:
   - it makes sense,
   - it uses an appropriate 'voice' for the task/audience,
   - it answers the question/addresses the topic,
   - punctuation and spellings are correct.
2. Ask yourself – "Have I missed anything out? Is there anything I could do to make it better?"

It is always worth asking a friend or parent to read your work before handing it in – sometimes they can see something that is quite obvious to the reader, but not at all obvious to the writer (this is the case with very accomplished writers too!).

- making a timetable for doing different activities and subjects,
- devising a simple project planner that breaks down the overall task and sets mini-deadlines to complete set pieces of the project,
- reviewing progress frequently (half-termly or more often if necessary), and
- helping to keep different subject files organised so that time is used more efficiently and important information or work does not get muddled up or lost.

It is also important to be realistic about how much information can be 'crammed' during revision. Help the child by looking through past examination papers to divide the content into three areas:

- Essential
- Important
- Useful 'if there is time'

Metacognitive strategies are those that involve the pupil thinking about the study skills needed and how to develop them most effectively:

- What helps him to learn?
- What hinders him?

Consideration of preferred learning styles can be helpful:

- Are visual representations easier to 'fix' (e.g. mind maps)?
- Does colour help?
- Does listening to explanations/texts help – would tape recordings be useful?

If the pupil has to explain something to someone (a brother, sister, parent or grandparent) it may help him to understand and remember it better. Revision should consist of more than simply reading through notes and will be most effective when:

- it is active, e.g. converting notes from one form to another, changing written notes to mind maps, producing question and answer cards, copying diagrams and labelling them from memory,
- it is involved in creating meaning, e.g. using information to answer model questions,
- study periods are short but frequent.

Examination vocabulary

Teach children how to read common words used in examinations and explain what they mean. Build up the child's vocabulary by going through past papers and identifying examination words and common sentence structures. Poor readers are often thrown by words that are not difficult to read but carry very little information. For example:

'Solve 6+3'

The pupil may be very capable of working out the sum, but be completely thrown by the word 'solve'. As they progress through school, there is an ever-growing list of vocabulary that pupils need to be able to read and understand. A checklist is provided on pages 69 and 70 with spaces for the teacher or pupil to add definitions.

Special examination conditions

In cases of more severe dyslexia, it may be possible to apply for special conditions within the exam itself. This may be an extra time allowance for the pupil, use of a word processor, a reader or an amanuensis (a scribe). This usually requires a written request and an assessment report from an Educational Psychologist or appropriately qualified teacher. Assessment reports are only valid for two years. This is because the pupil may have improved and this would give an unfair advantage.

Teachers who have a recognised qualification in dyslexia or psychology can conduct an educational assessment. The examination boards have published a list of acceptable qualifications. This maintains an appropriate level of quality control. It ensures that candidates are not unfairly disadvantaged, nor are they given an unfair advantage.

The up-to-date list can be obtained from: http://www.aqa.org.uk/admin/p_special_4.html

Schools wanting to make special arrangements for pupils in SATs must notify an LEA representative who monitors the situation. Non-LEA schools should contact QCA. An Educational Psychologist's assessment is not needed for special arrangements for these tests.

Examination Boards for GCSE, GCE 'A' levels and GNVQ Examinations will require a current assessment report from an Educational Psychologist or from a teacher with specialist qualifications for identifying, assessing and teaching pupils with dyslexia. Schools may be required to pay LEAs for such assessments. The report may not have to be submitted, but must be available if required.

Summary
Organisation and planning skills can be supported by:

- parents helping to develop good habits and supportive routines,
- teachers helping with general organisation,
- teaching essay writing and thinking skills before writing starts,
- considering how to revise and plan coursework,
- learning the words used by examiners,
- asking for special examination conditions.

Copies of the booklets:
- *Key Stage 1 Assessment and reporting arrangements*
- *Key Stage 2 Assessment and reporting arrangements*
- *Key Stage 3 Assessment and reporting arrangements*

are available free of charge from the Qualifications and Curriculum Authority (QCA) Tel: 01787 884 444; Fax: 01787 312 950; Email: info@qca.org.uk and www.qca.org.uk

---

GCE, VCE, GCSE & GNVQ. Regulations and Guidance relating to Candidates with Particular Requirements. Issued by the Joint Council for General Qualifications. Available from the awarding bodies including:
- Assessment & Qualification Alliance (AQA) Manchester; Tel: 0161 953 1180
- Assessment & Qualification Alliance (AQA) Guildford; Tel: 01483 506 506

Examination Board websites
- Assessment and Qualifications Alliance (AEB, SEG and NEAB): www.aqa.org.uk
- Edexcel: www.edexcel.org.uk
- OCR: www.ocr.org.uk
- Northern Ireland Council for Curriculum Examinations and Assessment: www.cea.org.uk
- Welsh Joint Education Committee: www.wjec.co.uk

Examination wordlist

Word	What does it mean?
Accurate	....
Analyse/analysis	....
Approximate	....
Categorise	....
Cause (and effect)	....
Characteristic	....
Comment	....
Compare	....
Consider	....
Contrast	....
Critical/criticise	....
Data	....
Decide	....
Deduce	....
Define	....
Discuss	....
Distinguish	....
Effect	....
Essential	....
Evaluate	....
Examine	....
Extent	....

5

Factor ....

Function ....
....

Hypothesis/hypothesise ....
....

Illustrate ....
....

Interpret ....
....

Justify ....
....

Maximum ....
....

Minimum ....
....

Optimal ....
....

Organise ....
....

Outline ....
....

Predict ....
....

Process ....
....

Prove ....
....

Purpose ....
....

Reason ....
....

Relate ....
....

Review ....
....

State ....
....

Summarise ....
....

Synthesis/synthesise ....
....

Dyslexia and Mathematics

Dyslexia is usually seen as a literacy problem affecting reading and spelling. However, just over half of dyslexic learners have problems with maths (BDA M01, *Dyslexia, dyscalculia and mathematics,* September 2001).

Maths is a symbolic language and pupils who have problems with letters may find numbers just as hard to recognise and recall. Those who have problems with orientation of 'b' and 'd' may find '6' and '9' equally problematical, and the difference between '11.92' and '119.2' may be missed by someone who has weak visual skills.

Learners may experience difficulties with all or some of the following areas:

- number recognition
- place value
- attaching meanings to symbols
- the language of mathematics
- recognising patterns

Some dyslexics may be slower at some aspects of maths than other children, but equally there are many dyslexics who excel at maths and can do the most convoluted calculations in their heads or appear to pluck numbers out of the air. Those who do well at maths may have strong concepts of numbers and awareness of patterns whereas pupils who fail are reliant on imperfectly remembered number bonds and may be further impeded by short-term memory problems. However, a great deal comes down to attitude. A pupil who has been encouraged to think of maths as fun – who connects it with birthdays, sport, or making and measuring things – is likely to be far more able to cope with the rigours of writing it all down than one whose main experience of maths has been restricted to drill and practice activities.

Of course, the first challenge is to get children to engage with maths. Some have good avoidance techniques and prefer to opt out rather than risk revealing how little they know. Let's look at some of the problems.

Number and notation

Naomi is 9 and is still counting on her fingers.

This may not be a problem. It may be that she needs reassurance and favours a tactile approach. There are a number of essential skills that need to be checked:

- Can she count?
- If you start with 21, can she count on to 30?
- Can she count backwards (21, 20, 19)?
- Does she know that 21 is bigger than 19?
- Does she understand that 121 is over 100?

Where pupils have problems with these basic concepts, a range of approaches can be employed to help them develop mathematical skills.

> Sam visualises numbers and their shape by thinking of a picture, so '4' is a house with 4 windows.

Concrete examples are often very helpful if used in conjunction with the written symbols they represent. As with the teaching of literacy, the approach should be multisensory: blocks should be examined visually, touched, and moved about in space. For example, if base ten blocks or coins are used, the operations of adding, taking away, etc. can be demonstrated in concrete terms. This is easier for dyslexics than having to deal with two-dimensional symbols on paper.

Pupils need to find what works for them.

> Oliver had difficulty in recognising the difference between the numbers '24' and '42' and confused similar 'pairs' of numbers. He used a red pen to write the tens and a blue pen for the units and remembered numbers by visualising the colours rather than their position.

Some pupils cope well with small numbers but once they are over 100, the system falls apart. Learners with dyslexia often need additional visual or tactile support to embed concepts.

Language and symbols

Once numbers are mastered, we move to symbols and operations. Symbols can be a source of difficulty. Not only are - and ÷ confusingly similar in appearance, but each can be expressed in a variety of ways: 'subtraction' may be expressed as 'less', 'minus' and 'take away'.

'12 take away 7' is the same as 'take 7 from 12', but the pupil may have problems identifying which number is taken from which and how it should be written.

12 divided by 4 may be expressed as:

- 4 divided into 12
- $12 \div 4$
- $\frac{12}{4}$
- 12 shared between 4

All mean the same thing, but learners may not realise this.

The skill of interpreting the special language of maths word problems needs to be taught carefully so that pupils can work out exactly what sort of number operation is needed:

'5 girls have 4 toys each. How many toys are there altogether?' (multiplication)

'If Nadim runs for15 minutes and William runs for 5 minutes less, how long has William been running?' (subtraction)

Children must be able to recognise *when* to multiply two numbers in a problem and *which* two numbers should be multiplied; that only comes with an increased understanding of mathematics and what you are trying to do. The Numeracy Strategy suggests that learners be allowed to make up their own word problems from number statements. Doing this can help the dyslexic understand the language of mathematics and how it is translated into formulae.

Quite a lot of teachers make a symbol sheet or, even better, get the pupils to make their own as they go along so that each symbol is associated with particular vocabulary. It gives the learner a chance to practise the symbols and to have a prompt that they can refer to. The symbol sheet that Michael built up over a period of time, as he came across particular phrases, is shown on page 74.

Number bonds and learning tables

Again, look for visual and tactile approaches. Use puzzles, games, construction equipment, calculators and software to help with number bonds and tables.

The BDA have a really helpful information sheet, which can be downloaded from http://www.bda-dyslexia.org.uk/d09maths/index.htm

It shows tips and hints for the 9 and 11 times tables, and how to draw a table square that is a ready reckoner for tables. By giving pupils a quick and easy guide to tables on paper you are supporting those who learn visually – learning by rote is an auditory method.

Calculators

Ofsted recently produced a report based on inspectors' observations of maths lessons and discussions with pupils in 68 schools. They expressed concern at the limited use of calculators.

"Despite its value the calculator is not a regular feature in the teaching of the

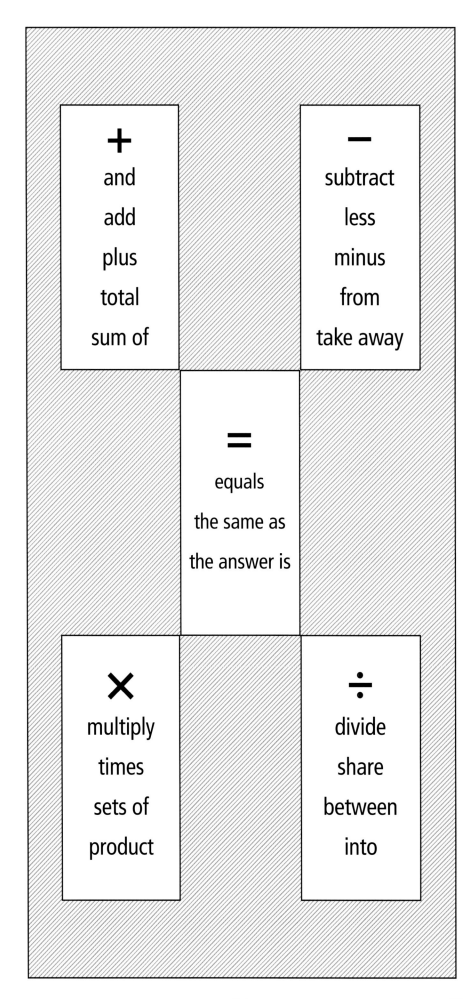

+
and
add
plus
total
sum of

−
subtract
less
minus
from
take away

=
equals
the same as
the answer is

✕
multiply
times
sets of
product

÷
divide
share
between
into

daily mathematics lesson at Key Stage two (pupils aged seven–11). A significant number of teachers refer to its use but do not give it enough emphasis. When it is used, teachers give too little attention to encouraging a range of options, such as using mental methods... alongside the calculator.”
(*Teaching of Calculation in Primary Schools A report by HMI*, April 2002, HMI 461)

Of course, a calculator is no substitute for good teaching, but some learners find that a calculator has proved a useful aid, not just to getting an individual answer right but, through repeated use, to learning particular products or number bonds.

Sofia can't tell the difference between '4005' and '405'. She writes '405' as '400' then adds on the '5' (4005).

Sofia's teacher needs to check if she knows the difference between hundreds and thousands and whether the problem is with the concept or just the notation (how it should be written). Sometimes a talking calculator can provide a breakthrough. Sofia would type in '4005' and it says 'four thousand and five'. This lets her know at once that she has got it wrong. The alternative is that she hands in her work to the teacher, waits for it to be marked and then gets it back a few days later, when she has forgotten what she was doing. The calculator is a tool in helping her take responsibility for her own learning.

Patterns

Sometimes learners work so slowly that they never discover patterns or make sense of what they are doing. They don't always realise that a particular exercise contains increasingly complex examples of the same type of activity. Using a calculator to practise number bonds or place value can be helpful. Many teachers and parents think that using a calculator is cheating, but it can help pupils speed up and recognise patterns.

Gareth and Robert were using a calculator to learn about multiplying and dividing by ten. During the lesson they operated on more than twenty decimal numbers. They made tables in their books showing the starting numbers and the answers.

.315	3.15	31.5
5.6	56	560
11.27	112.7	1127
0.05	0.005	0.0005

When they had discovered the rules, they predicted the answers for a few more numbers and used the calculator as a check. Then they added extra columns to their table and kept trying different sums, exploring multiplication and division by 100, 1000 and other powers of 10.

Without the calculator, Robert and Gareth would probably have spent the entire lesson doing six calculations and getting two of them wrong! There is no possibility that they would have discovered any pattern.

Estimation

Reasoning is the basis of estimation and a problem solving approach. These are skills that are just as important as basic knowledge. In fact, they may be even more crucial for those with specific learning difficulties since they may help them to overcome problems with memory, transferring skills and assimilating information.

Estimating and checking are vital skills for everyone, but they are especially significant for this group of learners who are often accustomed to being wrong and can easily become discouraged. Motivation can be a real problem with a learner who is intelligent enough to realise that they are underachieving and yet cannot find a way to improve their skills. By estimating answers they can begin to take some measure of responsibility for their own work.

These skills need to be developed in various ways: some pupils need a carefully structured programme of moving from the simple to the complex. For others a breakthrough seems to occur when real life parallels are used.

> Adrian is trying to work out 98 miles at 34.2p per mile. He uses a calculator and comes up with 3351.6. He writes down £3351.6 but then realises that no one would claim that much money for a car journey. This helped him to see the point of estimating. "Nearly 100 miles; 100 pennies in a pound so it's nearly £34."

Ways of working

It is often thought that dyslexic learners are not 'poor learners' but 'quick forgetters'. The National Numeracy Strategy may be helpful to them in a number of ways:

"The structure of the NNS provides frequent returns to topics allowing pupils to review and reinforce previous learning. Dyslexic pupils will greatly benefit from opportunities to overlearn. However, asking them to produce answers quickly, either mentally or written, will disadvantage most dyslexic learners." (BDA M01, *Dyslexia, dyscalculia and mathematics*, September 2001)

The whole emphasis for pupils with dyslexia needs to shift from writing to doing, from memorising to understanding, from looking to touching and moving.

- Let them learn by doing and then learn how to write it down.
- Make use of pictorial representation, number lines, table squares for number concepts and counting.

- Don't impose solutions; discuss what works for them and find ways of building on it.
- With older learners, make sure that the materials are appropriate to their age and interests.
- Link skills to real life situations, simulations based on shopping, catering or travel, for example.

> Gary had problems remembering different topics if he had not worked on them for a few weeks. Revision was a nightmare because he seemed to be approaching topics for the first time, often with limited success! He found that a small notebook with a worked example for each topic, which he could refer to every week, helped to keep the subject in his head.

It is essential to minimise verbal explanations. If the learner is given a sequence of spoken instructions before carrying out a task, he can be doubly handicapped. First, short-term memory may be at fault so one instruction may be omitted and secondly, since sequencing is a problem, he may get the order wrong.

Possible solutions:

- Let the pupil write down each step as he finishes it.
- Provide a scribe to write down what a pupil is doing, for future reference.
- Provide a written set of notes prepared by the teacher.
- Encourage the child to practise each step until it is embedded in his memory.

> Siobhan is quite competent at maths now but was always in the remedial group at school. She realises that the main problem was the way new topics were introduced.
> "The teacher would explain it and give us an example on the board. If I didn't understand, he would come and explain it again. I could always follow the first bit but got lost somewhere in the middle. He would explain it 3 or 4 times and each time he'd phrase it a bit differently. In the end there was a great fog of words in my head and I still didn't know what I was supposed to do. He'd say, 'Do you understand it now?' and I'd say, 'Yes, thank you.' I was too embarrassed and too confused to go through it again."

6

What about a computer program?

Generally, the computer can help in the following ways:

- It is associated with enjoyment.
- It provides a welcome change in presentation.
- It does not criticise, nor condemn.
- It has endless patience.
- It can provide extensive practice in numeracy skills.
- It can do many basic calculations, especially using spreadsheet, graph and statistics programs.
- It can improve presentation.

Programs need to be selected with care, taking into account the pupil's age, the presentation of the program and the level(s) and topics of work available.

Software may help both in the classroom and at home, but beware of using software just 'because it is fun'. Similarly, tedious drill and practice is still tedious if it is on screen.

Some programs such as *Intellimathics* are good tools for developing investigations about numbers. It has sorting activities and counting boxes with base ten blocks. Pupils move and manipulate objects, so it is a bridge between handling counters and coins on a table and the more abstract skill of writing down numbers on a piece of paper. Pupils move the mouse around the screen and, in some cases, this helps them to concentrate. Many programs work on a 'what if…' basis. 'What if I double the number?' 'What happens when I change the figures in this spreadsheet?'

It is not possible to suggest software for each topic and stage here, so use these guidelines to make an informed choice.

Choosing software
- Does it teach or provide practice and over-learning?
- Do the tasks test understanding rather than just memory?
- Does it have rewards or penalties, and if so are these a useful feature or a distraction?
- Are there visual cues on the screen to help learners work out answers?
- Are the screens clear and uncluttered?
- Is it clear what the learner has to do?
- Is there audio support?
- Does it need high-level literacy skills?
- Does it provide a chance to explore and experiment? Does it encourage a 'what if…' approach?
- With older learners, make sure that the materials are appropriate to their age and interests. Using software with pictures of toys just adds insult to injury!

Summary
- Maths is a symbolic language.
- Pupils may have problems with digit and symbol recognition.
- Not all dyslexic learners find maths difficult; some excel in this area.
- It can be useful to minimise verbal explanations.
- Try a range of approaches. Let the pupil move and manipulate objects, use colour, learn by doing and then learn how to write it down.
- Get pupils to make their own symbol sheets.
- Use a calculator to speed up work and to reinforce patterns.
- Remember that estimating and checking are vital skills.
- Beware of using software just 'because it is fun'; make sure it teaches skills instead of merely providing tests.

Emotional Support

The emotional needs of a child with dyslexia are just as important as, if not more important than, academic development. Some parents worry that the frustrations of not being able to deal with print or to record ideas will lead to depression and to an increased risk of:

- being bullied,
- strong feelings of inadequacy,
- feelings of failure,
- feelings of shame and embarrassment,
- suicide.

Charlton (1992) suggests that the emotional response of the child will become more significant with age. The experience of failing to read leads to demotivation or emotional blocking. This in turn leads to the child avoiding reading and reduces the expenditure of effort and persistence in trying to read. This then leads to a reduction in reading experience and less success compared to peers. The child sees the gap between themselves and their peers appear to get wider, and this increases their emotional response further eroding self-esteem.

The cycle continues, leading to what Stanovich (1986) calls the Matthew effect: good readers get comparatively better while poor readers get comparatively worse. Poor progress for SpLD pupils in secondary schools in reading development has been attributed to poor self-esteem, low self-confidence and experience of failure with literacy in primary schools (Ofsted, 1999). This means that the emotional impact of dyslexia cannot be ignored. In some studies, working on self-esteem through counselling has been shown to be more effective in improving reading skills than spending the same time on remedial teaching (Lawrence, 1985).

A number of emotionally supportive strategies are discussed throughout this book. In this section, we will consider understanding emotional responses and particular techniques to support specific emotional responses.

Emotional responses

Our emotional responses in any situation depend upon how we interpret what is happening around us. This in turn depends upon our previous experiences. If dyslexic children have a history of struggling with reading then it is not surprising to find that they often react quite strongly when presented with a reading task. The way in which they interpret the presenting task will affect the type and strength of emotion that they experience. This in turn will help to determine how they behave.

7

SUPPORTING CHILDREN

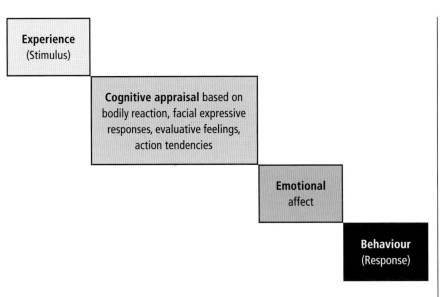

**Figure 3:
Thoughts precede
emotion and
emotion precedes
behaviour
(Squires, 2001b,
2002)**

The appraisal of the situation happens very quickly and we are often not aware of the contributing thoughts. Such thoughts are referred to as automatic thoughts and lead to the activation of a whole range of responses (see Figure 4).

Jane is asked to read out in class. An automatic thought flashes through her head so quickly that she is unaware of it, "I'm useless at reading". Her physiological system becomes activated with an increase of heart rate and release of adrenaline – the fight or flight hormone. Cognitively she thinks, "I'll probably make mistakes and the other kids will laugh". She becomes motivated to avoid the situation, "if I get sent out I won't have to do this". Emotional responses might include feeling ashamed or even angry that the teacher is putting her through this ordeal. She may even think that the teacher hates her – why else would she make her feel like this? Further evaluations of the situation might lead her to notice David smiling. Another automatic thought enters play, "he's laughing at me". This leads to the behaviour – verbal or physical abuse of the child who smiled. This is the behaviour the teacher sees and Jane is sent out of the room.

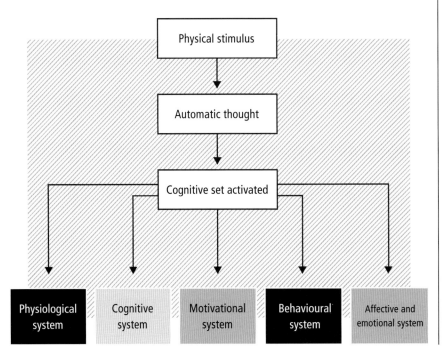

**Figure 4:
Cognitive set
activation
(Squires 2001b.
2002a)**

The child can be supported by helping them become aware of automatic thoughts. The relevance of the automatic thought to the current situation can then be checked out and alternatives offered. *What else could David have been smiling at? Perhaps he was laughing at you, perhaps he was pleased to see you were chosen. Maybe, he was smiling at the girl behind you. Perhaps he was pleased because the teacher had just said how pleased she was with his reading.* The child is taught to ask a series of questions to check out their response:

- How do we know which possibility is true?
- How can you find out? What evidence can you get?
- How would you feel in each case?
- How strongly?
- What would you do in each case?

Emotional blocking

Emotional blocking occurs when a task is presented that is well within the child's ability but the child considers it to be too difficult and reacts against that possibility by withdrawing from the situation. These strategies will help pupils to deal with the emotional blocking that leads to their reluctance to work through a problem or answer a question:

- Encourage risk taking with prompts to the child, e.g. 'have a go', 'what's your best guess?'
- Encourage risk taking in the classroom ethos, e.g. modelling that it is okay to make mistakes.
- Ask pupils to rate their confidence in knowing the answer. Then ask them for their answer and then for their rating again. If their answer is correct, use feedback to challenge the pupil's low self-evaluation. For example, "you gave yourself 2/10 for being sure that was the right answer – and your guess was right!"
- Use bridging techniques. For example, ask the pupils to think of other examples where they have known the answer – "this is a bit like the problem with the sinking and floating… what happened when I put the wood in water? How might that help us here?"
- Spend some time on class exploration of problems that have no 'right' answer to show that there are several possibilities rather than simply right or wrong.

Encouraging pupils in the search for solutions

Strong emotional responses such as anger and frustration are expressed by some pupils when things seem to be out of their control. Other pupils respond by withdrawing or apparently giving up. Engaging pupils in the search for solutions to perceived difficulties is helpful because it starts to bring the situation more into their control.

7

Open-ended questions

An open-ended starting point can be found by asking pupils how things might be different. Some children find this type of phrasing difficult and might find other open-ended questions easier, such as:

A genie appears and grants you three wishes. What would you ask for?

Once the pupil has started to express what he would like to be different, the task then becomes one of trying to create the steps to get there. How many solutions can you generate?

Paul: *I wish that I could read.*
Teacher: *You wish you could read better?* [Reframe and reflect]
Paul: *Yes.*
Teacher: *If it happened tonight, what would you read tomorrow?* [Make the discussion specific]
Paul: *Lord of the Rings*
Teacher: *Wow! That's a big book – lots of people like that. Who might help you?*

This discussion might then lead into a number of possible solutions:

- paired reading with a more able peer,
- an apprenticeship approach with a parent,
- whole class reading of the text,
- work on particular parts of the text with a teaching assistant,
- looking at an illustrated version, or
- making a personal version using a computer to write key phrases and adding drawings to make it into a book.

Rating scales

A simple scale of 1 to 10 (or 1 to 100) can be used to ask a pupil to identify the degree of a problem in different situations or over time. For example, Steven has problems with his work, he often does not complete the task set. He is asked to rate each subject:

Teacher: *On a scale of 1 to 10, 10 being really good and 1 being terrible, tell me how much work you are able to do in each subject.*
Steven: *English 5; Maths 4; PE 10; Science 5; History 8; Geography 1…*

Once this task is completed, there can be a focus on the subjects that have low scores:

Teacher: *What makes geography so difficult that it only scores a 1?*
Steven: *There's too much writing. I get lost when I am copying.*

The search for solutions then continues by looking at those subjects that score higher.

Teacher: *What happens when you are copying in Science?*
Steven: *The teacher gives us a worksheet and I can put my ruler under the*

words that I have to write – I don't get quite so muddled and don't have to keep checking where I am up to.

Teacher: *And in history – you gave that a high score – what helps there?*

Steven: *Well, the teacher tells us to do the work, then she comes round to make sure we're all doing it. Sometimes, when we copy off the board, she writes each line in a different colour. Often we have a sheet to stick in our books and we just fill in the gaps or write the answers to the questions.*

A number of solutions start to become apparent:

- having the target text near to where Steven is copying allows him to use his ruler as a tracking aid,
- different coloured writing on the board helps with tracking,
- sticking worksheets into his book helps him keep up, and
- being checked on helps him to start the work and not waste time at the beginning of the task.

With the last point, Steven could be empowered to help him engage with self-checking. He could be encouraged to see how well he can start his work in each lesson. A simple self-rating scale could be used for him to write onto photocopies of his weekly timetable:

1 – took ages to start; 5 – so-so; 10 – started straight away

Transitions

Transitions are simply changes from one class to another, from one school to another, or from one Key Stage to another. Transitions and change always provoke anxiety. This is natural; we all feel like this to some extent as we move from the safety of what we know and are comfortable with, towards the unknown and unpredictable. Parents and children have many worries about what might happen or might not happen. The key transition that all pupils make is from primary school to high school and this often causes the most worry for parents.

Some secondary schools have started to run summer schools for pupils who are transferring and who might have a weakness in literacy or numeracy. The intention is to provide additional teaching so that pupils are better able to cope with the secondary school curriculum and organisation.

Preparing for change

Preparation for moving to secondary school should start early on in Year 6. The primary school and secondary school are likely to have established procedures that will make the transfer of information efficient. The main problem will be that parents may not have decided on their choice of secondary school at this stage. The first task for parents is to visit possible secondary schools in order to make that decision during the autumn term.

Callum is due to transfer to the High School in September. His mother is quite concerned that this placement will not succeed. She is worried that:

- he won't be able to read the text,
- the pace of work will be much faster,
- the level of work will be much harder,
- it is a big school and teachers will not know him as well as they do in his small primary school,
- he will not be able to find his way around,
- he will forget what to take with him each day,
- there will be a lot of writing to do,
- he won't be able to cope with tests and exams, and
- homework will be difficult.

7

As part of the initial visits, parents should seek out key people who will be able to support their child:

● SENCo
● Head of Year
● Form Tutor (if known at this stage, though this is not normally decided until the summer term)

During the spring and summer terms further visits can be made to the school. Try to visit the secondary school when the school is working so that you and your child can:

● experience what lessons look like,
● see the range of work done (practical as well as writing),
● experience the vastness of the secondary school building,
● experience the crush in the corridors at break time,
● look to see where things are (e.g. toilets, break facilities, clubs, canteen), and
● meet key people again so that the child will have a friendly face they can turn to.

All of this is important in reassuring the child that his basic needs will be met and enabling him to look forward to starting at the new school.

During the summer term, link teachers from each school meet and share important information about special needs and strategies used to support the pupil. Many schools operate a system of visits for the pupils transferring so that they can spend some time with their new teachers and become familiar with the school layout. In some schools, incoming pupils are paired with pupils already in Year 7 and a pen-pal relationship is nurtured. This can be especially valuable if two dyslexic pupils can get together to share concerns and insights.

Some secondary schools have screening procedures for pupils entering the school. These may include reading tests, spelling tests and verbal and non-verbal reasoning tests to help identify children with special educational needs (including high ability), and provide a useful baseline against which to measure progress. Pupils with dyslexia may need to be reassured about these tests if they are not to constitute a bad start to secondary education.

Bullying

Some children are worried about bullying, and there may be many myths about what will happen to the new Year 7 pupils in September. It is a reality that bullying occurs in all schools (and in many workplaces). All schools are required to have established policies for dealing with bullying. Some schools have other strategies to help and these include:

- buddy systems – where older pupils befriend new pupils, usually in a structured way at first. In some schools, pupils are identified as 'buddies' on a rotational basis and will be available to pupils at break times or lunchtimes.
- peer mentoring systems and peer counselling systems – which operate in some schools where older pupils have received training from organisations such as Relate.

When parents are worried about potential bullying they should:

- work on past experience – if their child was not bullied at primary school then there is no reason to suppose that they will necessarily be bullied at secondary school. If they were bullied at primary school then how was the problem resolved? How will that help to resolve issues that might arise in the future (if they arise in the future)?
- talk to teachers at the secondary school to see how they might be able to help. They may have more specific resources to help, e.g. some schools now have trained counsellors.

Summer schools

Summer schools are run by some secondary schools and aim to improve basic literacy and numeracy. They provide a number of other opportunities:

- a chance to get to know some of the school staff before the pressure of term starts. Most primary school teachers are female and the move to a secondary school will provide some pupils with their first encounter of male teachers. This can have a positive effect by providing a male role model in a school setting.
- a chance to start to develop advanced study skills such as:
  - mind mapping,
  - note taking, and
  - working with ideas when writing, planning, reviewing and editing.
- time for school familiarisation, which is made easier when the school is almost empty, 'orienteering' games and map-making activities, which are useful preparation for the start of term.
- time for games to encourage:
  - team building,
  - thinking skills,
  - problems solving skills, and
  - for improving co-ordination (brain gym).
- teaching children strategies for everyday organisation, and encouraging good habits, e.g. spot prizes for having a pencil, ruler and eraser.

7

Summary

Emotional difficulties arise from a variety of sources and can lead to demotivation, emotional blocking or even more extreme reactions when a child is faced with print.

- Understanding how these emotional responses arise can help parents and teachers work with the child to overcome them (or even prevent them in the first place).
- Pupils can be encouraged to search for solutions as equal partners using open-ended questions and rating scales.

Transitions are a particularly difficult time for parents and children alike. They can be made easier through:

- adequate preparation for change,
- good links between key staff,
- summer schools.

7

The Parents' Role

For many parents, it comes as a great shock when their child fails to make satisfactory progress in reading at school. Often the child has been good with language in the home and has learnt to speak early. Many dyslexic children have been very articulate and have picked up and used words and phrases that are way beyond their years. They have enjoyed being read to and have a good memory for the fine details of stories.

Harry was a bright child who learnt to speak early. He was articulate and funny and picked up and used words and phrases which were way beyond his years. He enjoyed being read to and had a good memory for the fine details of stories. He loved *Dear Zoo* and *Mrs Plug the Plumber* and would join in, shouting: "Send for Mrs Plug!… When Mrs Plug was sent for, Mrs Plug came." He loved songs and rhymes and often recalled catch phrases from television programmes or the refrains of songs he had not heard for some months.

Harry had no problems with memory, no learning disabilities and had a love of the intricacies of language. His mother noticed that he did not recognise written words as quickly as his older sister, but reassured herself that every child is different and Harry would soon catch up when he got to school.

Like many children, Harry looked forward to going to school and his parents had no particular anxieties. He was bright and sociable and had enjoyed playgroup and nursery. When parents see their child's friends coming out of school with higher level reading books however, a certain unease or competitiveness creeps in. Why are they forging ahead? They think: "Perhaps if my child spent more time reading and less time watching TV, he would be as good." So before long there is the nightly battle over reading. The child begins to sense he is not quite up to the mark and wants to avoid the issue, the parents are determined to help the child to catch up. Progress is minimal or even non-existent and everyone in the house is sick of reading the same text night after night. Sometimes the child knows the book off by heart but cannot recognise the individual words out of context. He has an excellent memory but whatever is happening, it's not reading. A deficit model sets in. Instead of the child being known as the one who is funny, or good at football or who has a great singing voice, he begins to be known as the child who cannot read, who is a problem and a worry to his parents. It doesn't have to be like this. On page 89 we will start to look at what parents can do. Before that, let us take a moment to look at other aspects of the same problem.

8

The disaffected child

As the child gets older, he realises that he is in a special group, often with children who are not good at learning in general. What they come to realise however, is that they can have a good time together and the more outrageous they are, the more they make other children laugh. Here is something they are good at.

Girls are just as likely to have dyslexia as boys, but boys are far more likely to be identified for special help in schools. It is unclear why this is the case, but one factor may be the perception of reading and writing as a 'girly thing' and the ensuing lack of interest by boys. If girls take more of an interest in books and stories, playing at post-offices and writing in their Barbie diaries, the foundations of literacy skills are already being built. In most cases, they will have strong role models of mums and grans reading to them, writing shopping lists and sending notes to the teacher. This gender stereotyping is reinforced in primary schools where most of the staff are women. Reading can become a female occupation in the eyes of some boys. Their teachers and their mother seem to have an obsession with reading and writing and doing well at school. Girls take trouble with their work and produce nice neat projects, go to the library and find information, but boys play football, or hang out with their mates and try to get by. As time goes on, it seems more of an uphill struggle; they will never get there so why bother? Sometimes children hang on to this mind-set and, before long, they are getting into trouble at school and trouble on the streets, and in adolescence end up with a criminal record. Young offenders' centres and prisons have a disproportionately high number of dyslexic inmates. Sometimes the child follows a different route and becomes very dependent and clingy, constantly seeking reassurance and telling everyone he meets that he is dyslexic.

Sometimes, in an attempt to protect and support their children, parents unintentionally exacerbate the problem. One young man told me that his parents arranged after-school sessions with a private tutor and Saturday morning specialist classes. His diet was carefully regulated as they had heard about the effect of E numbers on concentration. No squash, no crisps, no sweets, no birthday cake or treats that other children enjoyed. He saw his lack of reading skills as his parents' problem. He functioned perfectly well without being able to spell; he disliked reading and saw it as a waste of time when he could be out on his bike or going fishing.

"Boys lag behind in early literacy skills and later on in English. The gap is apparent as pupils enter school for the first time and remains sizeable throughout pupils' primary schooling and into the secondary stages." Recent Research on Gender and Educational Performance, 1998, The Stationery Office.

Young offenders' centres and prisons have a disproportionately high number of dyslexic inmates. Dyslexia affects between 4–10% of the population. 52% of the randomly selected offenders showed strong indications of dyslexia. *The London Offender Study,* 1996.

Your child with literacy difficulties

What can you do?

First of all, try to stay calm and avoid making it an issue. Think to yourself, "Is this a real problem or might my child catch up?" Talk to teachers at the school. Sometimes parents have unrealistic expectations and compare their own child unfavourably with the most talented readers and not with the average child, so they over-react. Of course we all want our children to excel but not every child is a bookworm – some will have talents in languages or mathematics, sport or art. Many children develop skills relatively late, so if a child is not a fluent reader at the age of 6 it is not necessarily time to worry. Be guided by your child's teacher who will alert you to any concerns she may have about lack of progress. Schools usually begin to plan support strategies for a child when, after several terms in school, he demonstrates any or all of the following difficulties. He:

- cannot recognise and remember early 'key words',
- has difficulty in writing his own name correctly from memory,
- does not identify the 'initial sounds' of words. For example, he cannot say that 'baby' begins with a 'b', or cannot play 'I spy',
- cannot pick out an 'a' or 's' from a selection of plastic letters,
- finds it hard to re-form simple words made of plastic letters, when the letters are jumbled up (e.g. 'sit', 'mat', 'pig').

As children get older, many schools use reading ages (RA) as a measure of progress. As a rule of thumb they take a RA of two years less than chronological age (CA) as an indication of significant difficulty. (If a child is nine years old and has a RA of seven, he would usually be identified for extra support.) The tests used to establish a RA can give differing scores however, and it is often better to trust an experienced teacher's assessment – especially with young children. (See Table 2 on page 20.)

At the end of Key Stages, reading and writing will be assessed by SATs (Standard Assessment Tasks) in a way that compares each child with his peers and against the 'norm'.

Reading

Read together. This might sound obvious, but many parents spend time hearing their child read their reading book night after night but do no other reading together. Get the school book out of the way in ten minutes. It needs short, regular practice but it is not the most motivating reading activity. Choose books from the library together. Don't worry if the book your child chooses looks babyish – it is his choice. Similarly, if the book is too hard for him to read,

8

you can read it together. Try a bit of paired reading each day. Either you read a sentence and then your child reads the next one, or you read out loud together so that he can hear the words as he looks at them (see the guide on page 91).

Paired reading can be a delicate process with older readers. They will benefit from the practice but care should be taken not to make them feel 'babyish'. They may prefer to use non-fiction books – perhaps tied in with a homework task or lesson content. Poetry can be a good choice, especially when humorous, and has the advantage of being in short, manageable 'chunks'.

Talk about the story. So often, reading can become just a 'decoding' exercise where you work out each word but don't get the whole picture. Talk about what you have read during the day so that reading is seen as a normal activity and not a big hurdle which your child cannot overcome. As your child gets older and begins to read silently, try to read the same book as them from time to time. It takes only a short amount of time to read a slim children's paperback and will give you an opportunity to discuss the story with your child, what you (and he) liked and disliked about it, etc. This is an excellent motivator for developing readers – if an adult takes the time and trouble to read a book then it must be worth reading. Having one-to-one time together is also a reward in itself – especially if the discussion is kept light-hearted and fun.

Keep reading to your child. If he enjoys 'classics' such as *Treasure Island*, or is hooked on *Harry Potter*, these books are not easy reads. Reading to him will help him to finish the story in a reasonable time and keep up his interest. Many children enjoy being read to long after their transition to secondary school. Buy, or borrow from the library, story tapes (talking books) and encourage your child to play them on his personal stereo while waiting at the bus stop or travelling in the car.

Paired reading

- Start with the book closed. Make sure your child holds the book, or place it on the table in front of him, rather than you 'having ownership'.

- If this is a new book, ask your child what they think the story is about. Look at the title and the author. If it is a picture book, you may look at some of the pictures before starting to read – this will create a context for the story and 'cue-in' the reader.

- If you are continuing to read a book, ask your child: "What happened last time?"

- You may need to gently remind him of the storyline. Use this time to set up some expectations – "What do you think will happen?"

- Specific questions can be used to link previous reading with the new reading and pull the story together.

- Now open the book and read quietly together.

- Sometimes, you will take the lead. Sometimes, your child will lead.

- If your child struggles with a word, do not worry. Simply count to five in your head then tell him the word. The pause should give him a chance to work it out, but not be so long that it disrupts the flow of the story, or makes him feel embarrassed.

- Make a mental note of words that were difficult and use these (another time) for word-building practice or precision teaching.

- At the end of the reading, close the book and ask the child a few questions to see how much he has understood and remembered.

- Ask him what he thinks might happen next, what he would do if he was the main character, etc.

- It can be valuable to give the child an opportunity to re-read a passage from time to time. Having practised the text and worked out any difficult words, the re-reading gives him a chance to practise fluency and expression – and to enjoy it! This works especially well with dialogue, where the reader can concentrate on the 'voices' and have some fun.

8

Writing

If you have a computer, get your child to use it. Make posters, put on borders and experiment with fonts. Make it fun.

See if your computer will talk. If you have a sound card and can hear the sound effects on CD-ROMs, your computer has the capability to support synthetic speech. The easiest way to do this is to buy *textHELP: Read and Write 2000,* which sits on top of Microsoft Word and can be set up to read out loud as you type, or to read the whole document. It also provides full screen reading of text, menus and icons. Be prepared for your child to type in lots of rude words to start with as the computer will read anything! However, the novelty wears off quite quickly. Children can also copy entries from CD-ROMs or web pages and get them read aloud so they improve their listening skills and auditory memory, learning to get information from the spoken word.

textHELP!® Systems Ltd
Enkalon Business Centre
25 Randalstown Road
Antrim
Co. Antrim
BT41 4LJ
N. Ireland
Tel: 02894 428 105
Fax: 02894 428 574
http://www.texthelp.com
Also available from Semerc (www.semerc.com) and Inclusive Technology (www.inclusive.co.uk).

Quick writing projects

1. You are going to make the most disgusting pizza in the world. Write your shopping list.
2. Tales from Viking Days – choose a colour and font to make an attractive title.
3. Make a football poster.
4. Write a Valentine's Day card.
5. Produce a menu for your favourite meal.
6. Write a list of ten things you could not live without.
7. RED: make a list of all the things this colour suggests to you – sunsets, postboxes. Find the font colour tool. Write them all in red and choose a different font for each.
8. Camping in Wales, clubbing in Tenerife or safari trekking? Make a poster for your ideal holiday.
9. Devise a board game and write up the rules.
10. What wild animal would you choose to adopt? Use the web to find facts and pictures and write an appeal to be published in a magazine.

Spelling

Start with games:

- *Syllable spotting.* Many children have little idea of syllables. Explain that a syllable is a name for a beat. How many beats are there in these words: 'him', 'music', 'Superman'? Tell them each beat has at least one vowel ('a', 'e', 'i', 'o', 'u'). Sometimes, 'y' acts as a vowel (in words like 'my' and 'shy').
- *Word building.* Help them build phonic words (words that are spelt as they sound).

- *Use your word processor.* Make 'wordworms' like this –

ItwasadarkandstormynightwhentheshipsetsailfromDover

Get your child to use the space bar to put in the spaces. This helps with word recognition and reading.
- *Make 'word hunts'.* This is particularly useful when your child has lots of new vocabulary and spellings to learn. This is some of the vocabulary needed for history: burghers, gentry, nobles, serfs, peace, war, victory, defeat, treason, traitors, rebellion, riot, prisoners, punishments, branding, pillory, stocks, beheaded.

History 'word hunt' made with the SPA program.

SPA Ltd
PO Box 59
Tewkesbury
Gloucestershire
GL20 6AB
Tel: 01684 833 700

Use squared paper or, on the computer, make a grid in Word using *Tables*. Put in the words and then add extra letters around them, leaving some blanks if you need to simplify the task. Alternatively, you can buy a program called Word Square Maker from SPA which will do all the hard work for you and will create several different versions so the same words can be practised again and again.

Wordsearches can be fun, but some youngsters will find them laborious, so be guided by your child. Using lower case letters makes the words easier to recognise than using capitals.

Learning spellings for homework can be stressful for all concerned. Parents are anxious to 'do their best' for their child; the child is under pressure to perform and not let his parents down. The task itself can be boring and very difficult for a dyslexic child. All this and, at the same time, parents may have two or three other children to attend to, a meal to prepare and ironing to finish! The pointers on page 94 may be helpful.

If you find that learning spellings is taking a disproportionate amount of time and/or causing your child a lot of distress, it is worth speaking to his teacher or the school's SENCo about the problem. In some cases, a decrease in the number of words to be learnt will solve the problem. There is no reason why every child in class has to learn the same spelling list every week.

8

If you are working on spellings:

● Keep it short – ten minutes each night or in the morning four or five times a week is much more effective that forty minutes one night and half an hour at the weekend.

● Start a session with one or two spellings from the previous night/ week or words that you know the child will get right. This builds confidence.

● If there is a long list of words, split them up into one or two at a time: move on at the child's pace.

● Use a multisensory approach. Look at the word, say the word, break it up into syllables, single sounds or letter names – whatever works best for your child. Write the word – in the air, on each others' back, with your eyes closed and in joined-up writing if possible as this creates a tactile 'pattern'.

● Now ask your child to have a go at writing the word by himself, without a model.

● Is it correct?

● If it is – great celebrations! Pile on the praise. Come back to the word in ten minutes, then half an hour, then an hour – to practise and reinforce the spelling. This can be done in the commercial breaks, while washing-up, in the bath, etc. Be light-hearted about it.

● If your child is still having difficulty, ask him to spell as much of the word as he can and leave out the tricky bit. It can help to provide your child with the right number of letter spaces. For example, if the word is 'going', jot down the letter spaces _ _ _ _ _ then ask him to have a go: 'g o _ _ g'. "Well done, you're nearly there. Let's look at the tricky bit." In this case, you can say, "The missing letters spell a tiny word on their own, look 'in'. Let's practise them on their own. Now, put them into the bigger word." With more difficult words, a mnemonic might help (see page 100).

8

Secondary pupils

What about older children?

Some parents worry that their child will not cope at secondary school where they have new subjects, including modern foreign languages. They have to move from room to room, may have no class base, have to remember which books to take on which day, and deal with a variety of teachers.

Some parents transmit their anxiety to their children, so that far from the transition to big school being a time of excitement, it becomes an ordeal. In fact, many boys do better at secondary school. It seems as if they mature as more is demanded of them. Perhaps having male teachers makes a difference to their perception of school. Also, some of the secondary school curriculum has more 'boy appeal'. Many boys avoid drama and English but enjoy more practical subjects such as business studies, design and technology, ICT and sports. In 2002, 80,000 boys opted for GCSEs in PE, compared to only 37,000 girls. It may be that new subjects do not carry the taint of failure.

You can still work on spellings together. Many parents buy books of spellings but this is not necessarily helpful as they are likely to contain words the child will never use. You need to focus on words your child is already using. Look for the language they need for different subjects. Look in their exercise books and see which words are causing problems.

If subject-specific vocabulary is becoming a problem, you could ask the subject teacher for a list of words needed for a particular topic or term's work. Being able to prioritise these *in advance* of needing them will be a great benefit. Sometimes the teacher will be happy to provide a copy of the textbook for this purpose, though these may be in short supply in some schools. Alternatively, go through the SENCo who will be able to approach the subject teacher on your behalf – or even do a 'trawl' of several subject departments. Be patient! These are busy people, but should recognise the benefits that will come from taking the time to provide you with this information.

8

Jenny has a daughter Carla, in Year 8.

"She was getting more and more depressed about her spellings and her work always seemed to be covered in red ink. She used to write out the words over and over again using Look-Cover-Write-Check, but it didn't stick. If she didn't use the words for a few weeks, they would go again.

One night I went through her work and picked out about 50 spellings. Most of them were quite common words. Some of them had similar patterns so I put them together. We did 5–10 minutes each night after tea. I would write the word out correctly and we would talk about what she was getting wrong and how she could learn it. Sometimes we found a little word in a big word. She used to write 'tradgedy' but then we found 'rage' in the middle so she remembered that.

They were doing business letters at school. She used to put 'buisness' but when we talked about it and she saw it was from the word 'busy' – 'busi' + 'ness' – it made more sense. She couldn't write 'sincerely' but when we split it into 'since' + 'rely' and talked about how you rely on a sincere person, she got it. I realised that a lot of the time she made haphazard guesses about words. Once she could link a spelling to other words she knew, she got on much better.

These little 'tricks' worked for Carla but probably wouldn't work for another child. You have to know the child really well to find the things that work. That's where it helps if you are family because you have so many shared experiences you can tap into."

Summary

- Get out more! Try to develop a range of interests that you and your child can enjoy together which do not focus on reading and writing.
- Make sure your child has opportunities for physical activity. Some parents report that sport – especially swimming or dancing seems to improve reading skills.
- Consider diet, but don't be over-cautious. Provide a good balanced diet with plenty of fresh foods, but also the range of chocolate, crisps, etc that other children are allowed.
- Read to your child and try paired reading instead of insisting on your child reading to you. Take turns or read together so the child hears and sees the words.
- Make writing fun. Use the design features on a word processor. Make the computer talk. Let your child see you writing – and having to look up spellings from time to time.
- Don't lose sleep over spellings! Play Scrabble and other games. Make jokes about awkward words. Help your child to come to terms with his difficulty, while working on ways for him to improve.
- Take your time. Little and often is the best recipe. Stop if tempers get frayed. Try for ten minutes, five times a week as this shows the best results.
- Encourage independence. Help your child to do things for themselves and then stand back and let them try it out. Every time they organise themselves, they become more confident. If they fail, you should not take over but discuss how they can do better next time.
- Stay positive! Easier said than done, but do try. Do not hover anxiously, make negative comments or show that you think your child will fail.
- Find something to praise your child for – every morning and every evening.

Dyslexia and Me

When you were told you were dyslexic, how did you feel? Were you worried that you'd never be any good at reading and writing? Were you relieved because it explained why you had problems? Were you delighted because it meant you were gifted? Not many people see it as a gift at first. They have been told for so long that they are bad at things and can't keep up with the class – but this doesn't have to be you!

Look at this list of famous and talented people. They built on their strengths and took the world by storm. Obviously having problems with the written word didn't hold them back.

Entertainers	Poets	Actors
Cher	W.B. Yeats	Tom Cruise
Whoopi Goldberg	Benjamin Zephaniah	Dustin Hoffman
Eddie Izzard		Steve McQueen
		Jack Nicholson
		Anthony Hopkins
Writers	**Musicians**	**Film directors**
Hans Christian Anderson	John Lennon	Quentin Tarantino
Agatha Christie	Beethoven	Walt Disney
	Mozart	Steven Speilberg
Inventors	**Politicians**	**Sportsmen**
Albert Einstein	Winston Churchill	Carl Lewis
Henry Ford	Benjamin Franklin	Duncan Goodhew
Thomas Edison	John F. Kennedy	Jackie Stewart
Alexander Graham Bell		Magic Johnson
Leonardo da Vinci		

SUPPORTING CHILDREN

These people found what worked for them. They had imagination and an ability to think and do things in a different way. That's what made them stand out from the crowd.

Recognising your difficulties

Is this you?

- Some days, language is no problem, but on other days you can't put your ideas into words.
- You probably talk better than you write.
- Sometimes you read but don't get any meaning from it.
- You 'drift off' while reading.
- You may have lots of different spellings for one word.
- You're not good at proof reading because you don't spot that what you've written is not what was in your head.
- When you listen you don't get a sense of what is said; and you have problems coping with more than a couple of instructions at a time.
- You can get words in the wrong order when speaking.
- You have problems organising yourself and your time.
- You often turn up with the wrong equipment for lessons.

What can you do about...?

Organising yourself

- *Imagine yourself doing things.* If you have swimming tomorrow, imagine getting your swimming gear out of a drawer or the airing cupboard, wrapping it in a towel, finding a comb and shampoo and putting the whole lot in a bag. The more detailed the picture, the more likely you are to do it.
- *Have a large plastic box with a lid* to keep vital documents in. This becomes more important as you get older and have to keep track of chequebooks, letters, university applications, forms and your driving licence.
- *Make lists.* You don't have to write in words, you could use pictures or symbols. It saves you cluttering your mind with trivia.
- *Repeat things.* When someone gives you a list of instructions, say them out loud and in your head. Sometimes hearing your own voice can help to fix them in your mind.
- *Use 'Post-it notes'* to jot down things you think of on the spur of the moment. Stick them to the wall or door if you cannot deal with them at once. If you are at school stick them to the inside of a folder or exercise book.
- *Buy some brightly coloured folders* in which you put handouts, etc. Try to pick colours that are linked to the subject in your head, e.g. green for geography because it's about the earth.
- *Pack your school bag the night before.* You forget less if you are NOT doing it at the last minute.

Left and right

● Hold up both hands as in the picture below. Look at the shape made by your thumbs and first fingers. The one that makes the shape of an 'L' is your Left hand. If this doesn't work for you, try wearing a Ring on your Right hand.

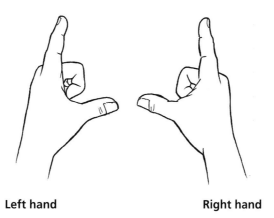

Left hand   **Right hand**

Reading

● *Read something every day* – even if it is the back of a cereal packet or an email. The more you read, the easier it will be for your eyes to cope with print.

● *Try out filters.* Ask your school if they have any. Try out different colours to see if they make reading more comfortable.

● *Ask your teachers to photocopy handouts onto different coloured paper* if this helps you.

● *Get a talking word processor* on your computer at home, if you have one. You can copy stuff off the Internet and CD-ROM entries into Word and it will read it out to you.

● *Get the video or audio tape* for books you are studying in English Literature. Watch or listen to the whole thing before you start reading. That way you will know the gist of the story and be able to take in more detail as you read.

Writing

● *Think about using mind maps for planning.* You can sketch them on a piece of paper or use a program like *Kidspiration* to create them. Look at these two pieces of writing about elephants. Which is easier for you?

- *Try to plan, then create, then correct.* If you worry too much about spellings in the early stages, you'll never write anything.
- *Record your ideas on tape,* if this helps.
- *Look at the design* of various pages, does the font used make a difference to you? Make your own set of samples by choosing different fonts – style, size, colour – on different coloured backgrounds. You can change the colour of the paper and the text very easily. Go to the *Format* menu on the Tool bar and click on *Background.* Choose the colour. Try these options:

- blue text on a yellow background,
- black text on a blue background, or
- red text on a blue background.

Spellings

- *Decide which words you want to learn to spell.* If you need them, and use them a lot, you are more likely to learn them.
- *Try to write the words.* Get a friend/parent/teacher to write the correct spelling at the side of your page. Pick out the part that you get wrong and write it in capital letters or in a bright colour. For example:

'yesterday'   'yesterday'   'yesTERday'

This helps you to notice the part you get wrong. Your eye is drawn to the correction and you are using your visual skills to remember it.

- *Develop mnemonics.* This is probably one of the hardest words to spell! It is pronounced 'nem-on-icks' and means 'an aid to memory'. For example, you can make up a sentence that spells a difficult word:

A right **i**diot **t**hought **h**e **m**ight **e**at **t**offee **i**n **c**hurch = arithmetic
Big **e**lephants **c**an't **a**lways **u**se **s**mall **e**xits = because

100

- *Find little words in big words,* e.g.

  'listen' = 'lis' + 'ten'
  'intermittent' = 'in' + 'term' + 'it' + 'tent'

- *Learn rules,* e.g. "after 'suc', 'ex' and 'pro', double E must go". This means that 'succeed', 'exceed', 'proceed' and 'precede' are all correct.
- *Use a cassette recorder.* Say the word, spell it then leave a pause. Listen to the tape as often as possible and repeat the spelling during the gap on the tape. After a while, the spelling will be second nature – as you think of the word, you will start reciting it.
- *Use a spell checker on your computer.* Look at the words it suggests. Keep a list.
- *Use a handheld spell checker* such as a *Franklin SpellMaster.* Type in your version of the word and see what it suggests.

Find out what you are good at

It is all too easy to get fed up and think that you will never overcome your difficulties. You might feel that your parents and teachers are only interested in your reading and spelling and are not interested in you as a person.

You can make some changes. Try to identify the things you are good at. No one can be good at everything. Tick the boxes on page 102 to show the things you are good at. Spaces have been left empty for you to write in your own ideas. You could ask people who know you to say what they think you are good at.

Summary
- Many famous people are dyslexic and gifted.
- Make sure you know and celebrate your strengths.
- Read something every day, even if it is just a cereal packet.
- Get organised. Use files and folders for school work and a large box for important documents.
- When you have a lot to remember, sit and think about what you need to do. Imagine you are doing it.
- Be colourful! Use coloured folders for different subjects. Try coloured overlays for reading. Use different background and text colours on the computer.
- Be active about spellings. What words do you need to know? How will you learn them? You can use look-cover-write-check; you can split word into syllables and exaggerate the sounds, you can look for little words in big words or you can develop your own silly sentences to help you remember.
- Be noisy! Say spellings out loud. Talk through what you are going to do and how you will do it. Use tape recorders to make voice notes or to practise composing. Use a computer with a talking word processor.

What am I good at?

Art and drawing	
Acting and drama	
Remembering information	
Discussing ideas	
Science and investigations	
Making friends	
Helping people	
Sport	
Speaking languages	
Singing	
Cooking and making up recipes	
Finding my way around	
Number work and maths	
Music	
Telling jokes	
Telling stories	
Playing computer games	
Looking after animals	
Spotting bargains in the shops	

Think about what you do well. How did you learn it? Can you apply this method of learning to other areas at school or at home? How do you want people to remember you? You need to show people what you are good at – if you don't tell them they won't know. Above all, celebrate all your successes, you've earned them!

9

References

The British Psychological Society (1999) *Dyslexia, Literacy and Psychological Assessment: Report of the Working Party* Leicester: BPS – Division of Educational and Child Psychology.

Brooks, P. and Weeks, S. (2000) *Individual Styles in Learning to Spell: Improving spelling in children with literacy difficulties and all children in mainstream schools* DfEE Research Report 108.

Bulstrode, C. and Hunt, V. (2000) What is mentoring? *The Lancet* **356**, 1788.

Charlton, T. (1992) Giving access to the national curriculum by working on the self. In Jones, K. and Charlton, T. (1992) *Learning difficulties in primary classrooms: delivering the whole curriculum* London: Routledge.

Cooper, P. and McIntyre, D. (1993) Commonality in teachers' and pupils' perceptions of effective classroom learning *British Journal of Educational Psychology* **63**, 381–399.

DfEE (Undated) *How can I tell if a child may be dyslexic? Handy Hints for Primary School Teachers.*

DfEE (2000) *Special Educational Needs: Special Edition (December 2000).*

Elliot, C. D., Smith, P. and McCulloch, K. (1996) *British Ability Scales (BAS-II) Administration and Scoring Manual* Berkshire: NFER. Note – the ability scores derived from the 2nd and 20th centile positions were used to find reading ages using the *BAS-II Achievement Scales Monthly Age Equivalents* tables.

Heaton, P. and Winterson, P. (1996) *Dealing with Dyslexia* London: Whurr.

Kelly, G. A. (1955) *The Psychology of Personal Constructs* New York: Norton.

Kullman, J. (1998) Mentoring and the development of reflective practice: concepts and context *System* **26**, 471–484.

Lawrence, D. (1985) Improving self-esteem and reading *Educational Research* **27** (3) 194–199.

Neale, M. D. (1997) *Neale Analysis of Reading Ability – Revised: Manual for Psychological Services* Windsor: NFER.

Nicholson, R. I., Fawcett, A. J. and Dean, P. (1995) Time-estimation deficits in developmental dyslexia – evidence of cerebellar involvement *Proceedings of the Royal Society of London. Series B-Biological Sciences* **259**, 43–47.

Nicholson, R. I., and Fawcett, A. J., Berry, E. L., Jenkins, L. H., Dean, P. and Brooks, D. J. (1999) Association of abnormal cerebellar activation with motor learning difficulties in dyslexic adults *The Lancet* **353**, 1662–1667.

Nleya, P. T. (1999) Perceptions of primary teacher educators on selected teaching skills *International Journal of Educational Development* **19**, 147–156.

Ofsted (1999) *Pupils with specific learning difficulties in mainstream schools: A survey of the provision in mainstream primary and secondary schools for pupils with Statements of Special Educational Needs relating to specific learning difficulties* London: Ofsted Publications Centre.

Ofsted (2000a) *Evaluating Educational Inclusion: Guidance for inspectors and schools* London: Ofsted Publications Centre.

Ofsted (2000b) *The SEN Code of Practice: Three years on. The contribution of individual education plans to the raising of standards for pupils with special educational needs* London: Ofsted Publications Centre.

Ofsted (2002) *The National Literacy Strategy: the first four years 1998–2002* London: Ofsted Publications Centre.

Rack, J. (1994) Dyselxia: The phonological deficit hypothesis. In Fawcett, A. J. and Nicholson, R. I. (Eds) *Dyslexia in Children: Multidisciplinary perspectives* Hertfordshire: Harvester Wheatsheaf.

Sawyer, C., Potter, V. and Taylor, T. (1994) Accessing the curriculum: How well do they need to read? *Support for Learning* **9 (3)** Oxford: Blackwell. Note – Fry reading scores have been converted to BAS scores using information in the article to make interpretation of assessment data easier.

Squires, G. (2001a) *An evaluation of a booklet of ideas to support teachers in reflecting about the strategies used when teaching dyslexic children* Unpublished research project submitted in part fulfilment of the requirements of the doctorate in educational psychology, University of Manchester.

Squires, G. (2001b) Thoughts, Feelings, Behaviour: Helping children understand themselves and take more control of their behaviour. *Special Children* Issue 134 (Jan. 01).

Squires, G. (2001c) Dyslexia Friendly. *Special Children* Issue 142 (Nov/ Dec. 01).

Squires, G. (2002) *Changing Thinking and Feeling to Change Behaviour: Cognitive Interventions* Ainsdale: Positive Behaviour Management.

Squires, G. (2003) *Cognitive Preferences and Spelling.* Unpublished research project submitted in part fulfilment of the requirements of the doctorate in educational psychology, University of Manchester.

Stanovich, K. (1986) Matthew effects in reading: some consequences of individual differences in the acquisition of literacy. *Reading Research Quarterly* **21**, 360–406.

Stanulis, R. N. and Russell, D. (2000) "Jumping in": trust and communication in mentoring student teachers. *Teaching and Teacher Education* **16**, 65–80.

Living by the word – even when you can't always read about it *The Guardian* 5 Nov. 98.

Treiman, R. (1997) Spellings in normal children and dyslexics. In Blachman, B. A. (Ed) *Foundations of Reading Acquisition and Dyslexia: implications for early intervention* New Jersey: Lawrence Erlbaum Associates.

Turner, M. (1997) *Psychological Assessment of Dyslexia* London: Whurr.

Wechsler Objective Reading Dimension (WORD) The Psychological Corporation.

Useful Contacts

- The Dyslexia Institute – Tel: 01784 463 851; www.dyslexia-inst.org.uk
- Becta – www.becta.org.uk
- The National Grid for Learning – www.ngfl.gov.uk
- British Dyslexia Association – Tel: 0118 966 2677; www.bda-dyslexia.org.uk
- The International Dyslexia Association – www.interdys.org
- Dyslexia Research Institute – www.dyslexia-add.org
- The Bristol Dyslexia Centre – www.dyslexiacentre.co.uk
- NASEN – www.nasen.org.uk
- www.dfes.gov.uk
- British Dyslexics – www.dyslexia.uk.com
- Dyslexia in Scotland – www.dyslexia-in-scotland.org
- dyslexia-information.com – www.dyslexia-information.com
- Barnaby Blackburn's personal site – www.iamdyslexic.com
- Dyslexia teacher – www.dyslexia-teacher.com
- Dyslexia parents resource – www.dyslexia-parent.com
- Dyslexia Research Trust – www.dyslexic.org.uk

Special CHILDREN

Supporting Children Series

The *Supporting Children* books are aimed at educational practitioners, both teachers and learning assistants, in specialist and non-specialist settings. Each book provides theory to inform the reader about a specific special need, while the main body of the text offers practical advice, support and activities to facilitate pupils' learning.

Supporting Children with ADHD

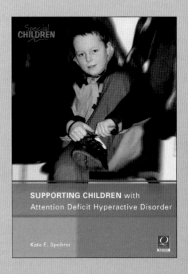

This book, with an introduction for teachers, is a photocopiable resource for children with ADHD. The activities and advice aim to enable these children to control their own feelings, thoughts and actions. By working through the activities, pupils will improve their self-esteem and understand their personality type.

Price: £15.00   **ISBN:** 1-84190-056-7   **Format:** A4 Approx. 88pp

Supporting Children with Autism in Mainstream Schools

It is increasingly common for children with autism to attend mainstream schools. Using the child-centred, whole-school approach provided in this resource, teachers will be able to implement strategies for supporting these children in the classroom, and successfully meeting their learning needs.

Price: £17.50   **ISBN:** 1-84190-055-9   **Format:** A4 Approx. 80pp

Supporting Children with Speech and Language Impairment and Associated Difficulties

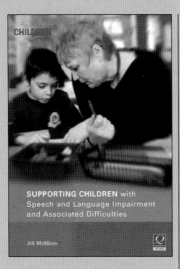

How do you identify and support pupils with speech and language impairment? This guide outlines the main areas of difficulty for pupils, and suggests how teachers can make the curriculum more accessible and so facilitate greater learning.

Price: £17.50   **ISBN:** 1-84190-083-4   **Format:** A4 Approx. 128pp

Supporting Children with Multiple Disabilities

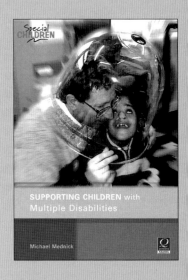

By following the practical framework provided, teachers will be able to implement a multi-sensory curriculum in the classroom. This will enable children with multiple disabilities to become more independent and active, and to develop effective communication skills.

Price: £20.00   **ISBN:** 1-84190-042-7   **Format:** A4 Approx. 180pp

Order form

I wish to place an order for the following titles:

Supporting Children with ADHD
£15.00

☐ copies

Supporting Children with Autism in
Mainstream Schools
£17.50

☐ copies

Supporting Children with
Multiple Disabilities
£20.00

☐ copies

Supporting Children with
Speech and Language Impairment and
Associated Difficulties
£17.50

☐ copies

PLEASE SEND MY ORDER TO:

Name: _____

Job title: _____

Delivery address: _____

_____

Postcode: _____

Tel: _____ Fax: _____

Email: _____

For Postage & Packing please add £3.00 U.K. £5.00 Overseas

☐ I enclose a cheque for £_____

made payable to The Questions Publishing Company Ltd.

☐ I wish to pay by credit card:

No. ☐☐☐☐ ☐☐☐☐ ☐☐☐☐ ☐☐☐☐ ☐☐☐☐

Expiry date: ☐☐☐☐   Signature: _____

Please give card address if different from delivery address:

_____

_____

Postcode: _____ Tel: _____

☐ I wish to pay by Official Order no. _____

**Credit Card Hotline
0121 666 7878**

Fax orders 0121 666 7879

Email sales@questpub.co.uk

Return completed form to
The Questions Publishing Company Ltd,
1st Floor, Leonard House,
321 Bradford Street,
Digbeth, Birmingham B5 6ET